Orthopaedic Word Book

Thomas J. Cittadine, MD

Springhouse
Word Book Series

Springhouse Corporation
Springhouse, Pennsylvania

Printed in the United States of America

Library of Congress Catalog Card Number: 88-42895

ISBN: 0-87434-419-0

SWB 7-010891

Preface

This book has been written primarily as a reference manual and spelling check for words, phrases, and surgical procedures commonly used in the fields of orthopaedics and sports medicine. These two areas encompass many disciplines including anatomy, biochemistry, biomechanics, engineering, genetics, immunology, medicine, microbiology, pathology, physics, prosthetics, physical and occupational therapy, research, surgery, and others. New terminology is constantly being generated even as this book is being written.

This book intends to integrate terminology from these different areas into a single reference. This book of terms should be useful to transcriptionists, secretaries, and technicians and also to those in areas such as nursing, physical therapy, and athletic training.

To my mother, Esther...
And in memory of my father, Lewis
November 20, 1912 to July 29, 1988

Acknowledgments

To Harry Benson for encouraging me to write this book and for his support during preparation.

To my office staff of Susie Smith, Sharyn Cruce, Curt McCarty, and Julie Brockhaus for their countless hours at the copy machine.

To my nephew, Michael C. Smith and to my good friends, Tom and Peg Langdoc for their excellent typing and computer skills and their patience in reworking the manuscript many times.

To my wife, Suzan who not only has assisted in preparation of the manuscript, but also has been supportive and patient during the period of preparation.

A

A.A.O.S. (American Academy
of Orthopaedic Surgeons)
A.O.S.S.M. (American
Orthopaedic Society for
Sports Medicine)
AML - (Anatomic Medullary
Locking Prothesis)
A or (Angstrom)
abacterial
abarthrosis
abarticular
abarticulation
abasia
abate
abatement
Abbott apparatus
Abbott approach
Abbott arthrodesis
Abbott and Carpenter approach
Abbott and Lucas approach
Abbott's method
ABD pads
abdomen
abdominal
abdominocentesis

abduct
abduction
abduction splint
abductor
abductor digiti minimi
abductor hallucis
abductor pollicis brevis
abductor pollicis longus
aberrant
aberration
ablate
ablation
abnormal
abort
abortive
above elbow (AE) amputation
above knee (AK) amputation
above knee suspension
abrachia
abrachiocephalia
abrasion
abscess
abscise
absconsio
absence

Additional Entries

absolute
absorb
absorbent
absorption
abstract
abuse
abut
abutment
A-C joint
A-C separation
acampsia
acantha
acanthesthesia
acceleration
accelerator
accessiflexor
accessory
accessory navicular bone
accident
accommodation
accretion
Ace bandage
Ace Colles technique
Ace Fisher frame
acellular
acentric
acephalobrachia
acephalopodia
acephalorhachia
acephalus
acetabular

acetabular index
acetabulectomy
acetabuloplasty
acetabulum
acetaminophen
acetone
acetylcholine
acetylcholinesterase
acheiria
acheiropodia
Achilles
    bursa
    jerk (reflex)
    tendon
achillobursitis
achillodynia
achillotenotomy
achondrogenesis
achondroplasia
achondroplastic
    dwarfism
achondroplasty
acid
acid phosphate
acid fast bacillus
acidophil
acidosis
acidosteophyte
aclasia
aclasis
acne

Additional Entries

A.C.O.S. - (American College of Osteopathic Surgeons)
acquired
acral
acrania
acrid
acroagnosis
acrobrachycephaly
acrocephalia
acrocephalopolysyndactyly
acrocephalosyndactyly
acrocontracture
acrocyanosis
acrodermatitis
acrodynia
acrodysplasia
acroedema
acroesthesia
acrohypothermy
acromegalic
acromegaly
acromelic
acromial
acromioclavicular
acromiocoracoid
acromiohumeral
acromion
acromionectomy
acromioplasty (Neer)
acromioscapular
acromiothoracic

acromyotonia
acro osteolysis
acroparalysis
acroparesthesia
acropathy
acrosclerosis
acrosyndactyly
A.C.S.M. - (American College of Sports Medicine)
ACTH (adrenocorticotropic hormone)
actin
Actinomyces
actinomycin
actinomycosis
actinoneuritis
active range of motion
active - assistive range of motion
activities of daily living (ADL)
activation
activator
actomyosin
acupuncture
acusection
acute
acyanotic
acyclovir
adactyly
adamantinoma
Adamkiewicz's artery
Adams ankle arthrodesis

Additional Entries

Acufex arthroscopic instruments

Adams' operation
Adams' saw
adaptation
adapter
Adaptic dressing
addict
addiction
Addis test
additive
adducent
adduct
adduction
adductor
adductor brevis muscle
adductor canal
adductor hallucis muscle
adductor longus muscle
adductor magnus muscle
adductor pollicus muscle
adductor tenotomy
adductor tubercle
Adelmann's operation
adenitis
adenocarcinoma
adenocellulitis
adenochondroma
adenochondrosarcoma
adenofibroma
adenoma
adenomyofibroma
adenomyosarcoma

adenopathy
adenosarcoma
adenosine
    3':5' - cyclic phosphate
    diphosphate (ADP)
    monophosphate (AMP)
    triphosphate (ATP)
adenovirus
adenylcyclase
adhere
adhesion
adhesive
adhesive capsulitis
adhesive drape
adhesive tape
adiadochokinesia
adiponecrosis
adipose
adjunct
adjustment
adjuvant chemotherapy
Adkins spinal fusion
ad lib.
adnexa
adolescence
adolescent
adrenal
adrenaline
adrenergic
adrenoceptor
adrenocortical

Additional Entries

adrenocorticotropin
Adriamycin
adromia
Adson forceps
Adson maneuver
adsorb
adsorbent
adsorption
adult
advancement
adventitia
adventitious bursa
adynamic
AE (above elbow)
aeration
aeremia
aerobic exercise
aerodermectasia
aeroembolism
aerogram
aerohydrotherapy
aerosol
afebrile
A-frame orthosis
afferent
affinity
afibrinogenemia
aftercare
agammaglobulinemia
aganglionic
agar

age
agenesis
agent
agglomerated
agglutination
agglutinin
aggressive
agility drill
aging
agitated
agnathia
agnosia
agraphia
AHF (antihemophilic factor)
AHG (antihemophilic globulin)
aid
AIDS (Acquired Immune
   Deficiency Syndrome)
ailment
ainhum
airplane splint
airsplint
airway
Akin procedure
akinesia
akinetic
ala (pl. alae)
Albee fusion
Albee graft
Albee shelf procedure
Albee's operation

Additional Entries

_____
_____
_____
_____
_____
_____
_____
_____
_____
_____

Albee table
Albers-Schönberg disease
Albert's operation
albicans
albinism
albino
Albert and Chase procedure
Albright synovectomy (hip)
Albright's syndrome
albumin
albuminemia
albuminuria
Albumisol
alcaptonuria
Alcock's canal
alcohol
alcoholic
alcoholization
aldehyde
aldolase
aldosterone
aldosteronism
aleukemia
algodystrophy
alignment
aliment
alimentation
alkali
alkaline
alkaline phosphatase
alkalosis

alkaptonuria
Allan procedure (calcaneus)
allantois
allele
allelism
Allen maneuver
Allen wrench
Allen test
allergen
allergy
allesthesia
alligator forceps
Allis clamp
Allis's sign
Allman classification (A-C joint)
Allman ankle reconstruction
alloantibody
allogeneic
allograft
allometric
allopathy
allopurinol
allotransplantation
alloy
Alm retractor
aloe
alopecia
ALRI (anterolateral rotarory
    instability)
ALS (amyotrophic lateral
    sclerosis)

Additional Entries

Allevyn decubitus care

alternating
alternation
aluminum foam splint
aluminum
Alzheimer's disease
A.M.A. (American Medical
Association; Australian
Medical Association)
ambu bag
ambulation
ambulatory
AMC wrist prosthesis
amebiasis
amelanotic
amelia
amelioration
amenorrhea
American Medical Association
(AMA)
American Orthopaedic
Association
American Orthopaedic Society
for Sports Medicine
American Society for Testing
Materials (ASTM)
amikacin sulfate
amino acids
aminoaciduria
aminoglycoside
aminopterin
ammonia

amnesia
anterograde
retrograde
traumatic
amnesic
amniocentesis
amnion
amniotic
amorphous
Amoss' sign
amoxicillin
AMP (adenosine monophosphate)
ampere
amphetamine
amphiarthrodial joint
amphiarthrosis
amphidiarthrosis
amphotericin B
ampicillin
amplification
amplifier
amplitude
ampule
amputation
Alanson's
Alouette's
amniotic
aperiosteal (Bunge's)
Callander's
Carden's
Chopart's

Additional Entries

amputation *(continued)*
- cineplastic
- circular
- congenital
- double flap
- Dupuytren's
- Farabeuf's
- Forbe's
- forequarter
- Gritti's
- Gritti Stokes
- guillotine
- Guyon's
- Hancock's
- Hey's
- hindquarter
- interscapulothoracic
- intrauterine
- Kirk's
- Langenbeck's
- Larrey's
- Le Fort's
- Lisfranc's
- MacKenzie's
- Maisonneuve's
- Malgaigne's
- open
- osteoplastic
- periosteoplastic
- Pirogoff's
- Ricard's

amputation *(continued)*
- spontaneous
- subastragalar
- Syme's
- Teale's
- traumatic
- Tripier's
- Vladimiroff-Mikulicz

amputee

AMRI (amtero-medial rotatory instability)

Amstutz and Wilson osteotomy

Amstutz total hip

amylase

amyloid

amyloidosis

amyoplasia

amyoplasia congenita

amyostasia

amyotonia

amyotrophy
- diabetic
- neuralgic

anabolic

anabolic steroids

anaerobe
- facultative
- obligate
- spore-forming

anaerobic

anal

Additional Entries

Amset ALPS (anterior locking plate system)

analgesia
  continuous caudal
  epidural
  infiltration
  permeation
  surface
analgesic
analgia
analogous
analogue
analysis
  qualitative
  quantitative
analyzer
Anametric knee prosthesis
anaphase
anaphylactic
anaphylaxis
anaplasia
anaplastic
anapophysis
Anaprox
anarrhexis
anasarca
anastomose
anastomosis
anatomic
anatomic neck
anatomic snuffbox
anatomy
  applied

anatomy *(continued)*
  artificial
  comparative
  descriptive
  developmental
  gross
  histologic
  macroscopic
  morbid
  physiological
  radiological
  regional
  surface
  surgical
  topographic
  x-ray
anchor
anchorage
ancillary
anconeal
anconeus muscle
anconitis
Anderson and Fowler osteotomy
Anderson and Green growth
  chart
Anderson and Hutchins
  technique
Anderson splint
Andre-Thomas sign
Andrew's operation
androgen

Additional Entries

androgenous
androsterone
anemia
anencephaly
anesthesia
    axillary
    Bier's local
    caudal
    endotracheal
    epidural
    general
    hypnosis
    hypotensive
    infiltration
    inhalation
    intercostal
    intraosseous
    intravenous
    local
    lumbar epidural
    parasacral
    paravertebral
    regional
    sacral
    spinal
    surgical
    topical
    transsacral
anesthesiologist
anesthesiology
anesthetic

anesthetist
anesthetize
aneuploidy
aneurysm
    abdominal
    aortic
    arteriovenous
    dissecting
    false
    fusiform
    infected
aneurysmal bone cyst (ABC)
aneurysmectomy
aneurysmoplasty
ANF (antinuclear factor)
Anghelescu's sign
angiitis
angina
angioblast
angioedema (angioneurotic
  edema)
angiofibroma
angiogram
angiography
angioma
angiomyolipoma
angiomyoma
angiomyosarcoma
angioneurotic
angioplasty
angiorrhaphy

Additional Entries

angle
angular
angular acceleration
angular displacement
angulation
anhidrosis
anion
anisocytosis
anisodactyly
anisokaryosis
anisomelia
anisotropic
ankle
ankle-foot orthosis (AFO)
ankylodactyly
ankylosis
    bony
    joint
    extracapsular
    false
    fibrous
    intracapsular
    surgical
ankylosing spondylitis (AS)
anlage
Annandale's operation
anneal
annular
annulus
anochromasia
anode

anomalous
anomaly
anonychia
anorchism
anorectal
anorectic
anorexic
anoxia
ansa cervicalis
anserine
antacid
antagonist
antalgic
antarthritic
antasthenic
antebrachium
antecedent
antecubital
anteflexion
antenatal
antephase
anterior
anterior cruciate ligament
anterior drawer test
anteroinferior
anterolateral
anteromedian
anteroposterior
anterosuperior
anteroventral
anteversion

Additional Entries

_____
_____
_____
_____
_____
_____
_____
_____
_____

anthropoid
anthropology
anthropometry
antiarthritic
antibacterial
antibiotic
antibody
anticholinergic
anticholinesterase
anticoagulant
anticonvulsant
antidepressant
antidote
antidromic
antiemetic
antifungal
antigen
antigenic
antigenicity
antihemolytic
antihemophilic
antihistamine
anti infective
anti inflammatory
antimicrobial
antineoplastic
antinuclear antibody (ANA)
antipyretic
antiseptic
antiserum
antistreptolysin

antithrombin
antitoxin
antivenin
antiviral
antivitamin
anuclear
anulus
anulus fibrosus
anus
anvil sign
A.O.P.A. (American Orthotics
    and Prosthetics Association)
aorta
    abdominal
    ascending
    descending
    thoracic
aortic stenosis
aortogram
aortography
apatite
Apert's disease (syndrome)
aperture
apex
Apgar score (scale)
aphalangia
aphasia
apical
aplasia
aplastic
Apley test

Additional Entries

apnea
apneic
apocope
apodal
aponeurosis
aponeurotomy
apophyseal
apophysis (pl. apophyses)
apophsitis
apparatus
appearance
appendage
appendix
appliance
applicator
apposition
apprehension
approach
approximate
apraxia
apron
A.P.T.A. (American Physical Therapy Association)
aqueous
A.R.A. (American Rheumatism Association)
arachnodactyly
arachnoid
arachnoiditis
Aran-Duchenne muscular atrophy (disease)

arc
arcade
arcade of Frohse
arch
arch supports
arciform
arcuate
ARDS (Adult Respiratory Distress Syndrome)
areflexia
areola
argentaffin
argon laser
arm
Armistead procedure
armpit
Armstrong acromionectomy
Arnold-Chiari deformity (malformation, syndrome)
arrest
arrhythmia
arterial
arteriectomy
arteriogram
arteriography
arteriole
arteriolosclerosis
arterioplasty
arteriosclerosis
arteriosclerotic
arteriospasm

Additional Entries

arteriostenosis
arteriostosis
arteriotomy
arteriovenous
arteritis
artery
arthragra
arthralgia
arthrectomy
arthritic
arthritide
arthritides
arthrocentesis
arthrochalasis multiplex
  congenita
arthrochondritis
arthroclasia
arthrodesis
arthrodynia
arthrodysplasia
arthroempyesis
arthroendoscopy
arthroereisis
arthrogram
arthrography
arthrogryposis
arthrokatadysis
arthrokleisis
arthrolith
arthrology
arthrolysis

arthromeningitis
arthrometer
arthrometry
arthroncus
arthroneuralgia
arthro-onychodysplasia
arthropathy
arthrophyma
arthrophyte
arthroplasty
arthropyosis
arthrorheumatism
arthrosclerosis
arthroscope
arthroscopy
arthrosis
arthrosteitis
arthrostomy
arthrosynovitis
arthrotomy
arthroxerosis
arthroxesis
articular
articulate
articulated
articulation
artifact
artificial
ascending
asepsis
aseptic

Additional Entries

Ashworth arthroplasty
A.S.I.F. (American Society of
  Internal Fixation)
Asnis cannulated screw
aspergillosis
Aspergillus
asphyxia
aspirate
aspiration
aspirator
aspirin (ASA)
asplenia
A.S.I.S. (anterior superior iliac
  spine)
assay
assistant
association
assortment
astasia
astereognosis
asternal
asthenia
asthenic
asthma
astragalectomy
astragalus
astringent
Astroturf
asymmetrical
asymmetry
asymptomatic

asynergy
atactic
atavism
ataxia
ATC (certified athletic trainer)
atelectasis
atelorachidia
atherosclerosis
athetoid
athetosis
athlete
athletic
athletic trainer
atlantoaxial
athetoid
athetosis
atlantoaxial
atlas
atmosphere
atonic
atony
atopy
Atosoy procedure
ATP (adenosine triphosphate)
ATPase (adenosinetriphophatase)
atraumatic
atresia
atrioventricular
atrophic
atrophied
atrophy

Additional Entries

Aston cartilage reduction system

atropine
attachment
Attenborough knee prosthesis
attenuation
attrition
atypical
Aufranc approach
Aufranc cup
Aufranc-Turner total hip
aurotherapy
auscultation
Austin-Moore prosthesis
autism
autoamputation
autoclave
autogenous
autograft
autoimmune
autoinfection
autologous
autolysis
automatic
autonomic
Autophor total hip

autoplasty
autopsy
autosome
auxiliary
AV, A-V, (arteriovenous.)
avascular
avascular necrosis
aviator's astragalus
Avila approach
avulsion
avulsion fracture
awl
Axer technique
axial
axilla
axillary
axillary block
axis
axon
axonotmesis
axoplasm
azathioprine
azygos vein

Additional Entries

_____
_____
_____
_____
_____
_____
_____
_____
_____
_____
_____
_____
_____
_____
_____
_____

Additional Entries

B

Babinski reflex, sign
Babinski-Frohlich syndrome
bacillus
bacitracin
Baciu and Filibiu ankle
　arthrodesis
back
backbone
backflow
back-knee
backscatter
bacteremia
bacteria
bactericidal
bacterioid
bacteriophage
bacteriostatic
bacteriotoxic
bacteriotoxin
bacterium
bacteriuria
Bacteroides
Badgley arthrodesis
Bado classification
Bahler elbow arthroplasty
Bailey and Dubow technique
Baker's cyst
Baker and Hill osteotomy

Baker procedure
Balacescu technique
balance
balanced suspension (traction)
Balkan frame, splint
ball
ball and socket joint
ball and socket osteotomy
ballet
ballistics
balloon
ballotable
ballottement
balm
band
　iliotibial
　Parham
　periosteal
bandage
　abdominal
　Ace
　Baynton's
　capeline
　circular
　compression
　crucial
　demigauntlet
　Desault's

Additional Entries

bandage *(continued)*
    elastic
    Esmarch's
    figure-of-8
    gauntlet
    gauze
    Genga's
    Gibney
    Hippocrates'
    plaster
    pressure
    Ribble's
    Richet's
    roller
    Sayre's
    spica
    spiral
    spiral reverse
    Theden's
    triangular
    Velpeau's
banjo cast
bank
Bankhart lesion
Bankhart repair
Banks and Laufman
   approach
Banks graft
BAPS (Biomechanical ankle
   platform system)
bar

Barr procedure
Barr-Record procedure
barbiturate
barbotage
barium
Barlow's disease
Barlow's test
barotrauma
barrier
Barsky technique
Barton's bandage
Barton's fracture
Barton's operation
Barwell's operation
basal
basal metabolic rate
base
baseball elbow
baseball finger
baseball splint
baseline
basement membrane
basicranial
basilar
basilic vein
basioccipital
basivertebral
basket
basket forceps
basophil
basophilic

Additional Entries

Barouk button space, → used for hallux valgus deformity
Barouk microscrew
Barouk microstaple.

Bassett electrical stimulation
   system
Batchelor technique
Bateman prothesis
bath
Batson's complex (veins)
battery
Bauer technique
Bauer, Tondra, and Trusler
   technique
Baumann's angle
Baumgard and Schwartz
   technique
Baumgartl dysplasia
bead (rachitic b's)
beaded
Beall, Webel, and Bailey
   technique
beam
beaver blade
Bechtol prothesis
Beckenbaugh technique
Becker technique
Beclard's amputation
Becton technique
bedfast
bedpan
bedsore
Beevor's sign
Bekhterev's (Bechterew's)
   arthritis

Bekhterev test
Bell's law, palsy (paralysis)
belladonna
Bell-Tawse technique
belly
Bence-Jones protein
bend
bending irons
bending moment
bends
benign
Bennett approach
Bennett dislocation
Bennett retractor
Bennett's fracture, operation
benzene
benzodiazepine
benzoin
Berger's method, operation
beriberi
Berman and Gartland technique
Bertolotti syndrome
Betadine
betamethasone
bevel
biarticulate
bicapsular
biceps
   brachii
   femoris tendon
bicipital

Additional Entries

_____
_____
_____
_____
_____
_____
_____
_____
_____

bicipital groove
biconcave
biconvex
b.i.d. (twice a day)
Bier block
Bier's amputation
bifid
bifurcate
bifurcation
Bigelow's ligament
bilateral
bilirubin
binder
binocular
bioceramics
biochemistry
biocompatible
biodegradable
Biodex machine
biodynamics
bioequivalent
biofeedback
bioimplant
bioingrowth
biologic
biomaterial
Biomechanical ankle platform
  system (BAPS)
biomechanics
biometric prothesis
biophysics

biopsy
  aspiration
  excisional
  exploratory
  incisional
  needle
  punch
  sternal
  surface
  surgical
  total
biorhythm
bipartite
bipedal
bipenniform
bipedicle
biplane
bipolar
bipolar prothesis
birefringence
birefringent
birth
birthmark
bivalve
bladder
  atonic
  automatic
  irritable
  neurogenic
blade plate
Blair arthrodesis

Additional Entries

Blair and Morris' technique
Blair and Omer technique
blastocoele
blastocyst
blastoderm
Blastomyces
blastomycosis
blastula
bleb
Bleck technique
bleeder
bleeding
bleomycin
blister
    blood blister
    fever blister
    fracture blister
    water blister
block
    axillary
    Bier
    caudal
    epidural
    field
    intercostal
    intraspinal
    paracervical
    paraneural
    parasacral
    paravertebral
    perineural

block *(continued)*
    presacral
    sacral
    stellate
    sympathetic
blockage
blood
blood bank
blood culture
blood group
bloodless
blood plasma
blood pressure
blood serum
blood type
Blount disease
Blount retractor
Blount blade plate
Blount technique
blue toe syndrome
Blumensaat's line
Blundell-Jones osteotomy
Blundell-Jones technique
blunt dissection
board certified
board eligible
Bobechko hook
body
body cast
body jacket
Boeck's disease, sarcoid

Additional Entries

_____
_____
_____
_____
_____
_____
_____
_____
_____

Bohler splint
boil
bolus
bond
bone
    brittle
    cancellous
    compact
    cortical
    lamellated
    woven
bone age
bone bank
bone block
bone density
bone graft
bone infarct
bone island
bone marrow
bone morphogenic protein
bone salts
bone scan
bone wax
booster
boot
    cast boot
    Gibney's
    Unna's paste
    walking boot
boot top fracture
Boplant

Bora procedure
Borden, Spencer, and Herndon
    osteotomy
border
Borggreve operation
Bose nail fold removal
boss (carpal)
Boston brace
Bosworth approach
Bosworth fusion
Bosworth procedure
Bosworth screw
Bouchard, nodes (nodules)
bout
boutonniere
boutonniere deformity
boutonniere repair
Bovie bipolar electrocautery
Bovie electrocautery
bovine
bowleg
bowler's thumb
bowstring
bowstring sign
Boyd and Anderson procedure
Boyd and McLeod procedure
Boyd and Sisk procedure
Boyd approach
Boyd graft
Boyd procedure
Boyes technique (transfer)

Additional Entries

_____
_____
_____
_____
_____
_____
_____
_____
_____

boxer's elbow
boxer's fracture
B.P. (blood pressure)
brace
bracelet test
brachial
brachial plexus
brachialgia
brachiocephalic
brachiocrural
brachiocubital
brachiocyrtosis
brachiogram
brachiotomy
brachium
brachybasia
brachycephalic
brachydactyly
brachymetacarpia
brachymetapody
brachymetatarsia
brachyphalangia
brachystasis
brachytherapy
bracing
Brackett technique
Brackett and Osgood Approach
Bradford frame
Brady and Jewett technique
bradycardia
bradykinesia

Brahams technique
brain
brain stem
branch
Brand technique
Brand tendon stripper
Brannon and Wickstrom
    technique
Braun technique
breadth
break
breast
breaststroker's knee
breech delivery
Brett technique
brevicollis
bridge
Brighton electrical stimulation
    system
brim
brisement
Bristow-Latarjet procedure
Bristow procedure
Brittain arthrodesis
Brittain and Dunn arthrodesis
brittle
brittle failure
broach
Brockman technique
Brodie's abscess
Brodie's disease

Additional Entries

Brodie's knee
Brodie's ligament
bronchogenic carcinoma
bronchoscopy
bronchospirometry
bronchus
Brooks and Jenkins fusion
Brooks and Seddon transfer
Broomhead approach
Brown-Adson forceps
Brown dermatome
Brown-Sequard syndrome
Brown technique
brown tumor
Brown and McDowell procedure
brucella
brucellosis
Brudzinski's sign (reflex)
bruise
bruit
Bruser approach
Bryan technique
Bryan and Morrey approach
Bryant's traction
bubo
Buchholz acctabular cup
Bucks extension, fascia
Bucks traction
Buck-Gramcko pollicization
buckling
bucket handle tear

Bucky diaphragm, rays
bud
Budd-Chiari syndrome (disease)
Buerger's disease, symptom
buffer
Bugg and Boyd technique
bulb
bulb suture
bulbocavernosus reflex
bulbus
bulla (pl. bullae)
bumper fracture
BUN (blood urea nitrogen)
Buncke technique
bundle
bundle branch block
Bunge's amputation
bunion
bunionectomy
bunionette
Bunnell procedure
Bunnell suture
Bunnell pull out wire
Bunnell test
bupivacaine hydrochloride
bur
Burgess technique
Burkhalter technique
Burman technique
burn
Burns plate

Additional Entries

burnishing
Burow's solution
burr (bur)
Burrow's technique
bursa (pl. bursae)
bursectomy
bursitis
bursocentesis
bursolith
bursopathy
bursotomy
burst
burst fracture

Burton's line (sign)
Bush technique
busulfan
Butazolidin
Butler technique
butt
butterfly fracture
buttock
button
buttonhole
buttress plate
bypass

Additional Entries

Additional Entries

cable graft
cable twister orthosis
cachectic
cacomelia
cadaver
café-au-lait spots
Caffey's disease
Caisson disease
Calandruccio nail
Calandruccio compression
   device
calamine lotion
calcaneal
calcaneitis
calcaneoapophysitis
calcaneoastragaloid
calcaneocavus
calcaneocuboid
calcaneodynia
calcaneofibular
calcaneonavicular
calcaneoplantar
calcaneoscaphoid
calcaneotibial
calcaneovalgocavus
calcaneus
calcanodynia
calcar

calcar femorale
calcareous
calcidiol
calcifediol
calciferol
calcific
calcification
calcinosis
calcipenia
calcitonin
calcitriol
calcium
calcium phosphate
calcium pyrophosphate
calciuria
calculus
Caldani's ligament
Caldwell and Coleman
   technique
Caldwell and Durham technique
calf
caliber
calibration
calipers
calisthenics
Callahan approach
Callander's amputation
Callaway's test

Additional Entries

_____
_____
_____
_____
_____
_____
_____
_____
_____

callosity
callous
callus
calor
calorie
calvarial
calvarium
Calve Perthes disease
cambium
Camite tendon transfer
Campbell and Akbarnia
   procedure
Campbell arthrodesis
Campbell graft
Campbell, Molesworth, and
   Campbell approach
Campbell's ligament
camptocormia
camptodactyly
camptomelia
camptospasm
Canadian hip prosthesis
Canadian Orthopaedic
   Association
canal
Canale technique
canaliculus
canalization
Can Am brace
cancelli
cancellous

cancellous bone graft
cancellous bone screw
cancericidal
cancerophobia
cancerous
Candida
candidiasis
cane
   adjustable
   English
   quadripod
   tripod
cannula
cannulate
cannulated nail
Cantelli's sign
cantilever fatigue
cantharidin
capacity
capeline
Capener technique
capillary
capital epiphysis
capitate
capitellum
capitulum
capsular
capsule
capsulectomy
capsulitis
capsulodesis

Additional Entries

capsuloplasty
capsulorrhaphy
capsulotomy
carbenicillin
carbide
carbocaine
carbohydrate
carbon
carbon dioxide (CO_2)
carbon dioxide (CO_2) laser
carbon fiber
carbuncle
Carceau and Brahms ankle
 arthrodesis
carcinogen
carcinoma
carcinomatosis
carcinomatous
Carden's amputation
cardiac arrest
cardiogenic shock
cardiogram
cardiologist
cardiopulmonary
cardiovascular
c-arm image intensifier
Carnes technique
Carnesale approach (hip)
carotid artery
carotid endarterectomy
carotid triangle

carpal
carpal boss
carpal tunnel release
carpal tunnel syndrome
carpectomy
carpitis
carpocarpal
carpometacarpal
carpopedal
carpophalangeal
carpus
carrier
Carroll arthrodesis
Carroll technique
Carroll and Taber arthroplasty
carrying angle
Carter-Rowe view
cartilage
cartilage-hair hypoplasia
cartilaginous
cartwheel fracture
case history
caseous
cassette
cast
cast boot
cast brace
cast sock
cast syndrome
casting
Castle procedure

Additional Entries

CAT (computerized axial tomography) scan
catabolic
catalyst
catecholamine
catgut
catheter
catheterization
cathode
Catteral classification
cauda equina
cauda equina syndrome
caudad
caudal
caudocephalad
causalgia
caustic
cauterizaion
cautery
Cave and Rowe procedure
Cave approach
cavernous
cavernous hemangioma
cavity
cavovalgus
cavovarus
cavus
c.b.c. (complete blood count)
CDH (congenital dislocated hip)
CE angle of Wiberg
Ceclor

cefaclor
cefadroxil
cefamandole
cefaparole
cefatrizine
cefazaflur sodium
cefazolin
ceforanide
cefoxitin
cell
cellular
cellularity
cellulitis
cement
cementless
cement gun
cement mantle
center
center of gravity
centigrade
centimeter
central cord syndrome
central nervous system (CNS)
central slip (tendon)
centrifugation
centrifuge
centriole
centromere
centrosome
centrosphere
cephalad

Additional Entries

cephalexin
cephalic
cephalic vein
cephalocaudad
cephaloridine
cephalosporin
cephalothin
cephapirin
cephradine
ceraceous
ceramic total hip
cerclage
cerclage wire
cerebellar
cerebellospinal
cerebellum
cerebral
cerebral palsy (CP)
cerebroside
cerebrospinal
cerebrospinal fluid (CSF)
cerebrovascular
cerebrovascular accident (CVA)
cerebrum
certified athletic trainer (ATC)
certified orthotist (CO)
certified prosthetist (CP)
cervical
cervical plexus
cervical rib
cervical spine

cervical traction
cervical vertebrae
cervicobrachial
cervicobrachialgia
cervicodynia
cervico occipital
cervicoscapular
cervicothoracic
cervicotrochanteric
Chaddock's reflex (sign)
Chakirgil technique
chalk bones (Albers-Schönberg)
Chamberlain's line
Chambers technique
Chance fracture
Chandler technique
channel
Chapchal technique
charcoal
Charcot's arthritis
Charcot joint
Charcot-Marie-Tooth atrophy,
  disease
charley horse
Charnley approach
Charnley arthrodesis
Charnley prosthesis (hip, knee)
Charnley retractor
Charnley-Mueller approach
Charnley-Mueller prosthesis
Chatzidakis implant

Additional Entries

CHAG (Coralline hydroxyapatite Goniopora)
bone graft substitute

chauffer's fracture
Chaves and Rapp transfer
Chaves procedure
cheilectomy
cheiragra
cheiralgia paresthetica
cheirarthritis
cheirobrachialgia
cheiromegaly
cheiroplasty
cheiropodalgia
cheirospasm
chemical
chemistry
chemolysis
chemonucleolysis
chemoprophylaxis
chemoreceptor
chemosterilized
chemosurgery
chemotaxis
chemotherapy
chest
    barrel
    flail
    funnel
    pigeon
Chevron osteotomy
Chiari-Arnold syndrome
Chiari osteotomy
chiasm

Chiene's operation
chilblain
Childress technique
childhood
chip fracture
chiropractor
chisel
chi-square
chlorambucil
chloramphenicol
chlorpromazine
Cho technique
cholecalciferol
cholecystectomy
cholesterol
cholinergic
cholinesterase
cholinoceptor
chondral
chondrectomy
chondrification
chondritis
chondroblast
chondroblastoma
chondrocalcinosis
chondrocarcinoma
chondroclast
chondrocostal
chondrocyte
chondrodynia
chondrodysplasia

Additional Entries

chondrodystrophia
chondrodystrophy
chondroepiphyseal
chondroepiphysitis
chondrogenesis
chondroitin
chondroitin sulfate
chondrolipoma
chondrolysis
chondroma
chondromalacia
chondromatosis
chondrometaplasia
chondromucoid
chondromucoprotein
chondromyxoid fibroma
chondromyxoma
chondromyxosarcoma
chondronecrosis
chondro-osseous
chondro-osteodystrophy
chondropathology
chondropathy
chondrophyte
chondroplasia
chondroplast
chondroplasty
chondroporosis
chondroprotein
chondrosarcoma
chondrosarcomatosis

chondroskeleton
chondrosternal
chondrosternoplasty
chondrotomy
chonechondrosternon
Chopart's amputation
Chopart's joint
chorda dorsalis
chorda-mesoderm
chordoma
chorea
     Huntington's
     Sydenham's
choreiform
choreoathetosis
Chrisman and Snook procedure
Christiansian procedure
Christian's disease (syndrome)
Christmas disease, factor IX
chromatid
chromatin
chromatin-negative
chromatin-positive
chromium
chromosome
chronic
chronology
chronologic
chrysotherapy
Chuinard technique (femoral
     osteotomy)

Additional Entries

Chuinard and Peterson technique
(ankle arthrodesis)
Chvostek's sign
Chvostek-Weiss sign
chymopapain
Cidex
Cincinnati incision
cineangiography
cineplastic amputation
cineplasty
cineradiography
cineroentgenography
Cintor knee prosthesis
ciprofloxacin
circadian rhythmn
circoelectric bed
circular
circulatory
circumduction
circumference
circumflex
circumscribed
cisplatin
clamp
Clark technique
Clark and Axer technique
clasmocytoma
classification
claudication
clavicle
clavicotomy

claviculus
clavipectoral
clavus
clavus durum
clavus mollum
clawfoot
clawhand
claw toe
clay shoveler's fracture
Clayton procedure
clear cell sarcoma
cleavage fracture
cleft
cleft lip
cleft palate
Cleland's ligaments
cleidocranial
cleidocranial dysostosis
Cleocin
Cleveland, Bosworth, and
Thompson pseudoarthrodesis
repair
click (Ortolani's)
clindamycin
clinic
clinical
clinodactyly
Clinoril
clinotherapy
Clinotron bed
clonus

Additional Entries

closed amputation
closed biopsy
closed reduction (fracture or
  dislocation)
closed suction irrigation
closed wedge osteotomy
clostridial
Clostridium
closure
clot
clothespin graft
Cloutier knee prosthesis
cloverleaf nail
Cloward procedure
cloxacillin sodium
clubbing
clubfoot
clubhand
cluneal
cluneal nerves
Clutton's joint
cm (centimeter)
CMC (carpometacarpal)
C.N.S. (central nervous system)
coagulate
coagulation
coagulator
coagulopathy
coapt
coaptation splint
coarctation

coat
coated carbon fiber
cobalt
cobalt-chrome
Cobb elevator
Cobb gouge
Cobb technique
cobra plate
cobra retractor
coccidiodes
coccidioidimycosis
coccyalgia
coccydynia
coccygeal
coccygectomy
coccyx
cock-up splint
codeine
Codivilla graft
Codman angle
Codman approach
Codman exercises
Codman sign
Codman triangle
coefficient
coefficient of friction
coenzyme
cogwheel sign
colchicine
cold intolerance
Cole pull out wire

Additional Entries

Cole procedure
Coleman procedure
Coleman and Noonan technique
Coleman, Stelling, and Jarrett
    technique
collagen
collagenase
collagenous
collapse
collar
collar button abcess
collarbone
collateral
collateral circulation
collateral ligaments
Colles fracture
collimator
Collis method
Collison plate
colloid
Colonna technique
Colonna and Ralston approach
colony count
Coltart arthrodesis
Colton classification
column
coma
comatose
comminuted
comminution
communicable

compact
compact bone
compartment
compartment syndrome
compatible
compensation
compensatory curve
complaint
complement
complex
compliance
complicated
complication
component
composite graft
compound
compound dislocation
compound fracture
compress
compression
compression arthrodesis
compression dressing
compression fracture
compression neuropathy
compression screw (nail)
compromised
computerized axial tomography
    (CAT scan)
concave
concavity
concavoconcave

Additional Entries

concavoconvex
concentric
concussion
conditioning
conduction
conduction time
condylar
condylar blade plate
condylar implant arthroplasty
condyle
condylectomy
condylocephalic nail
condylotomy
cone arthrodesis
configuration
conform
congenital
congenital anomalies
congenital bars
congenital dislocated hip (CDH)
congenital myotonia
congenital scoliosis
congenital torticollis
congenital vertical talus
congestive heart failure
conjoined tendon
Conn technique
connective tissue
connector
conoid ligament
Conray

conscious
conscious-sedation
conservative
constancy
constrained knee prosthesis
constriction
consultant
consultation
contact
contagious
contaminant
contamination
contiguous
continuity
contour
contract
contractile
contraction
contracture
contraindication
contralateral
contrast
contrast bath
contrast medium
contrecoup
control belt
control cables
contusion
conus
conus medullaris
convalescence

Additional Entries

convex

convexity

convolution

convulsion

Cooley's anemia, disease

Coonrad prosthesis

Coonse and Adams approach

Coopernail's sign

Cooper's ligaments

coordination

coracoacromial

coracobracialis muscle

coracoclavicular ligament

coracohumeral ligament

coracoid

coracoiditis

cord

    lateral

    medial

    posterior

    spinal

cordoma

cordotomy

core

core biopsy

core protein

corn

    hard

    soft

coronal

coronary

coronoid process

correction

correlation

corrosion

corrosive

corset

cortex (pl. cortices)

cortical

cortical bone

cortical bone graft

cortical defect

cortical desmoid

cortical fracture

cortical screw

corticocancellous graft

corticospinal

corticosteroid

corticotropin

cortisol

cortisone

Corynebacterium

cosmesis

cosmetic

costal

costalgia

costectomy

costicartilage

costicervical

costispinal

costochondral

Additional Entries

costoclavicular
costosternal
costotranverse
costotransversectomy
costovertebral
costovertebral angle
costovertebral joint
Cotel cast technique
Cotel traction
Cotton fracture
Cotton osteotomy
cotton roll
Cotton loader position
cotyloid
Couch, DeRosa, Throop
  technique
coumarin
counterbalance
counterincision
countertraction
couple
coupling
countersink
Coventry osteotomy
Coventry and Johnson
  classification
Cover Roll dressing
Cox technique
coxa
    magna
    plana

coxa *(continued)*
  valga
  vara
coxalgia
coxarthritis
coxarthrocace
coxarthrosis
coxitis
coxodynia
coxotomy
coxsackievirus
Cozen and Brockway z plasty
Cozen approach
C.P. (cerebral palsy)
CPK (creatine phosphokinase)
CPM (continuous passive
  motion)
CPR (cardiopulmonary
  resuscitation)
Cracchiolo forefoot arthroplasty
crack
cradle
Craig needle
Craig abduction splint
cramp
craniad
cranial
cranial halo
craniofacial
craniosacral
craniostenosis

Additional Entries

craniostosis
craniosynostosis
cranium
craterization
cravat
Crawford dexterity test
Crawford and Adams cup
c-reactive protein (CRP)
creatine
creatine phosphokinase (CPK)
creatinine
creatinine clearance
creep
creeping substitution
Crego closed reduction
Crego osteotomy
cremaster muscle
cremasteric reflex
crepitation
crepitus
crescent sign
crest
cretin
cretinism
cretinoid
crevice
cricothyroid
critical
cross-finger flap
cross-friction massage
cross-leg flap

cross-linking (collagen)
crossmatching
cross-reactivity
cross table lateral
crossunion
Crouzon's disease
CRP (c-reactive protein)
cruciate
cruciate ligaments, anterior and
  posterior
cruciate pulleys
cruciate screw
crural
crutch
Crutchfield tongs
Cruveilhier's atrophy
cryosurgery
cryotherapy
cryptococcosis
crystal
crystallization
crystalloid
C.S.F. (cerebrospinal fluid)
CT (computerized tomography)
Cubbins technique
Cubbins, Callahan, and Scuderi
  approach
cubital
cubital tunnel
cubitocarpal
cubitoradial

Additional Entries

Crescentic base wedge osteotomy

cubitis valgus
cubitis varus
cuboid
cuboid sign
cuff
culture
culture and sensitivity (C & S)
cuneiform
cuneocuboid
cuneonavicular
cuneoscaphoid
cup arthroplasty
curative
curet
curettage
curette
curettement
curie
current
Curtin technique
Curtis arthroplasty
Curtis technique
curvature
curve
curvilinear incision
Cushing's disease
cutaneous
cutaneous nerves
cutaneous stimulators
cuticle
Cybex machine

Cybex testing
cyclic loading
Cyriax technique
Cutter cast
CVA (costovertebral angle;
    cerebrovascular accident)
CVP (central venous pressure)
cyanosis
cyclophosphamide
cylinder
cylinder cast
cylindrical reamers
cyst
    aneurysmal bone
    Baker's
    bursal
    dermal, epidermal
        inclusion
    epithelial
    inclusion
    myxoid
    sebaceous
    solitary bone
    subchondral
    synovial
    unicameral bone
cystic
cystic fibrosis
cystinosis
cystogram
cystoscopy

Additional Entries

cytochrome c
cytology
cytoplasm

cytotoxic
cytotoxin

Additional Entries

D

dacron
dactylitis
dactylomegaly
Danlos' syndrome (disease)
dantrolene sodium
Darrach technique
Darrach McLaughlin approach
Darvon
Darvocet
Das Gupta procedure
d' Aubigne procedure
d' Aubigne prosthesis
daunorubicin
David technique
Davis arthrodesis (hip)
Davis graft
Dawbarn's sign
DCP (dynamic compression plate)
de Andrade and MacNab technique
Debeyre, Patte, and Elmelik technique
de Quervain's disease
de Quervain's release
dead
debridement
debris

debulking
Decadron
decalcification
decalcify
decay
deceleration
decerebrate
decompression
decompression laminectomy
decontamination
decortication
decubitis position
decubitis ulcer
decussation
dedifferentiation
deep
deep knee bends
deep palmar arch
deep peroneal nerve
deep tendon reflexes (DTRs)
deep transverse ligament
deep vein thrombosis (DVT)
defatted
defect
defective
deficiency
deficit
deformation

Additional Entries

deformity
degenerative
degenerative arthritis
degenerative disk disease
degenerative joint disease
degloving injury
degradation
degree
dehiscence
Dehne cast
dehydration
Dejerine-Landouzy dystrophy
Dejerine-Sottas atrophy, disease
Delbet hip classification
delayed flap
delayed primary closure
delayed union
deletion
Delorme exercises
delta
delta phalanx
deltoid
deltoid ligament
deltoid muscle
deltoid splitting approach
deltopectoral groove
demarcation
dementia
Demerol
demifacet
demigauntlet

demineralization
demyelinate
denarcotize
dendrite
denervate
denervation
Denis Browne bucket or tray
Denis Browne splint
Dennyson and Fulford
    arthrodesis
dens
density
dental drill
dentinogenesis imperfecta
denture
denudation
deossification
dependent drainage
depilatory
depolarization
Depo-medrol
deposit
depressed fracture
depression
depth gauge
derangement
Dercum's disease
dermabrasion
dermal
dermal fibromatosis
dermatin sulfate

Additional Entries

dermatitis
dermatoarthritis
dermatofibroma
dermatofibrosarcoma
dermatographism
dermatome
    Brown
    Padgett
    Reese
    Stryker
dermatomyositis
dermodesis
dermoid cyst
dermometer
dermoplasty
derotation brace
derotation osteotomy
Desault's sign
Desault's dislocation
descending
desensitization
desiccate
desmectasis
desmodynia
desmoid
desmoma
desmoplasia
desmoplastic
desmoplastic fibroma
desmorrhexis
desmosis

desmotomy
desquamation
destructive
detachment
detergent
detoxification
detritus
devascularization
development
deviation
device
devitalize
DeWar and Barrington
    procedure
DeWar and Harris procedure
dexamethasone
Dexon suture
dexterity
dextran
dextrose
Deyerle procedure, apparatus
diabetes
diabetic
diagnosis
diagnostic
diagram
dial
dial lock
dial osteotomy
dialysis
diameter

Additional Entries

Diamond and Gould technique
diaphragm
diaphyseal
diaphysectomy
diaphysis
diaplasis
diarthrosis
Dias and Gingerich technique
diastasis
diastematomyelia
diastrophic
diastrophic dwarfism
diathermy
Diatrizoate
diazepam
DIC (disseminated intravascular
  coagulation)
dicheiria
Dickson technique
Dickson and Dively technique
Dickson and Willien technique
didactylism
dietary
diethylstilbestrol
dietitian
differential
differentiate
diffuse
diffuse idiopathic sclerosing
  hyperostosis (DISH)
digit

digital
digital arteries
digital nerves
digital veins
digitation
dihydroxycholecalciferol
  (1,25-dihydroxyvitamin D)
dilatation
dilator
dimension
Dimon and Hughston procedure
dimple
DIP (distal interphalangeal)
DIP fusion
DIP joint
diphtheroid
diplegia
diplegic cerebral palsy
diplococcus
disability
disability rating
disarticulation
disc
discharge
discitis
discogenic
discogram
discography
discoid
discoid lateral meniscus
discopathy

Additional Entries

discrepancy
disease
disimpaction
disinfect
disinfectant
disintegration
disjunction
disk
diskectomy
diskitis
diskogram
dislocation
dismemberment
disorder
disorganization
disorientation
dispensary
displacement
disproportion
disruption
dissection
dissociation
dissolve
distal
distally
distance
distension
distortion
distraction
distress
diuretic

divergence
division
DLE (discoid lupus
    erythematosus)
DMSO (dimethyl sulfoxide)
DNA (deoxyribonucleic acid)
D.O. (Doctor of Osteopathy)
D.O.A. (dead on arrival)
dog ears
Doll method
Dolobid
dolor
dome fracture
dominant
donor
donor site
Doppler ultrasound
dorsal
dorsal bunion
dorsal column
dorsal hood
dorsal spine
dorsal vein
dorsalis
dorsalis pedis artery
dorsalis pedis pulse
dorsiflexion
dorsolateral
dorsolumbar
dorsomedian
dorsoradial

Additional Entries

DonJoy knee braces (one word, caps on D and J)

dorsoscapular
dorsoventral
dorsum
dosage
dose
dosimeter
dosimetry
double-action ankle joint
double-blind
double hip spica
dowel
dowel graft
Down's syndrome (disease)
doxorubicin
D.P.M. (Doctor of Podiatric Medicine)
drain
drainage
drape
draping
drawer sign
dressing
drill
drill guide
drill hole
drill point
driver-extractor
dropfoot
drop-lock ring
drug
drug addict

drug reaction
Drummond wire technique
du Toit staples
du Toit and Roux capsulorrhaphy
dual lock prosthesis
dual onlay graft
Dubinet prosthesis
Duchenne's disease
Duchenne-Erb paralysis, syndrome
Duchenne-Landouzy dystrophy
Duckworth and Smith technique
duct
ductile
ductility
dull
dumbbell
Dunlop traction
Dunn-Brittain triple arthrodesis
Dunn and Hess femoral component
Dunn and Hess osteotomy
Duocondylar knee prosthesis
Duopatellar knee prosthesis
Duplay's bursitis
duplication
Dupuytren's contracture
Dupuytren's disease
Dupuytren's fracture
dura
dural

Additional Entries

dura mater
Duran and Houser wrist splint
duraplasty
Durham plasty for flatfoot
duroarachnitis
Duverney fracture
DuVries procedure
dwarf
dwarfism
Dwyer and Wickham electrical
  stimulation system
Dwyer
    gouge
    osteotomy
    rod
dynamic compression plate
  (DCP)
dynamization
dynamometer

Dynaplex knee
dysarthrosis
dysautonomia
dyscrasia
dysesthesia
dysfunction
dysgenesis
dyskinesia
dynmelia
dysmetria
dysostosis
dysplasia
dysplastic
dysraphia, dysraphism
dystonia
dystrophic
dystrophy
dystropic

Additional Entries

Duran program

Additional Entries

E

Eaton prosthesis
Eaton-Littler technique
Eberle release
eburnation
eccentric
eccentric exercises
ecchymosis
ecchymotic
ECG (electrocardiogram)
ECRB (extensor carpi radialis brevis)
ECRL (extensor carpi ECRL: longus)
ectoderm
ectodermal
ectomorph
ectopic
ectopic ossification
ectromelia
ectrosyndactyly
ECU (extensor carpi ulnaris)
eczema
EDC (extensor digitorum communis)
edema
edematous
Eden technique
Eden-Hybbinette procedure

EDL (extensor digitorum longus)
EDQ (extensor digiti quinti)
EEG (electroencephalogram)
efficiency
effusion
Efteklar clamp
Efteklar technique
Egawa classification
Egawa sign
Egger's operation
Egger's plate
EHL (extensor hallucis longus)
Ehlers-Danlos syndrome (disease)
Eicher prosthesis
EIP (extensor indicis proprius)
elastic
elastic bandage
elastic modulus
elastic orthosis
elasticity
elastin
elastomer
Elastoplast
elbow
electric stimulation
electroanalgesia

Additional Entries

_____
_____
_____
_____
_____
_____
_____
_____
_____

electrocardiogram (EKG)
electrocautery
electrode
electroencephalogram (EEG)
electromyogram (EMG)
electromyography
electrophoresis
elephantiasis
elevator
Elliot plate
Ellis technique
Ellis-Jones procedure
Ellison procedure
Elmslie and Trillat technique
Elmslie ankle reconstruction
elongation
Ely's test (sign)
embedded
embolectomy
embolism
embolization
embolus
embryo
embryogenesis
embryology
embryoma
emergency
eminence
E.M.S. (Emergency Medical
    Service)
enamel

enarthrosis
en bloc
encapsulated
encephalitis
encephalography
encephalomyelitis
encephalopathy
enchondroma
enchondromatosis
enchondrosarcoma
enchondrosis
endarterectomy
end-artery
end to end anastomosis
end to side anastomosis
endemic
Ender nail
end-feet
endocrine
endocrinologist
endocrinopathy
endoderm
endogenous
endomorph
endomysium
endoneural ·
endoneurium
endoneurolysis
endoplasmic
endoplasmic reticulum
endoprosthesis

Additional Entries

end-organ
endorphin
endoskeletal prosthesis
endoskeleton
endosteal
endosteum
endothelial
endotheliosarcoma
endothelium
endotoxin
endotracheal
end-plate
end point
endurance limit
energy
Engelmann's disease
Engelmann's disk
Englehardt femoral prosthesis
enlargement
Enneking staging
enostosis
enteric coated
enterobacter
enterovirus
enthesis
entoderm   .
entrapment syndrome
enucleate
environment
enzyme
eosinophil

eosinophilia
eosinophilic granuloma
EPB (extensor pollicis brevis)
ependyma
ependymoma
epicondyle
epicondylitis
epidemic
epidemiology
epidermis
epidermoid
epidermoid cyst
epidermolysis
epidural
epidural block
epidural veins
epinephrine
epineurial neurorrhaphy
epineurium
epiperineurial neurorraphy
epiphyseal dysplasia
epiphyseal fracture
epiphyseal plate
epiphyses
epiphysiodesis
epiphysiod
epiphysiolysis
epiphysis
epiphysitis
epithelial
epithelialization

Additional Entries

epithelioid sarcoma
epithelioma
epithelium
epithelization
epitrochlea
EPL (extensor pollicis longus)
eponychia
eponychium
epoxy
Eppright osteotomy
equinocavovarus
equinocavus
equinovalgus
equinus deformity
Erb's point
Erb-Duchenne paralysis
Erdheim-Chester disease
erector spinae muscle
ergometer
ergonomics
Erickson, Leider, and Brown
  technique
Eriksson cruciate reconstruction
erosion
erysipelas
erythema
erythematous
erythrocyte
erythrocyte sedimentation rate
  (ESR)
erythromycin

erythropoietin
eschar
Escherichia coli
esmarch
Esmarch's bandage, tourniquet
E.S.R. (erythrocyte
  sedimentation)
Esser's graft
Essex-Lopresti classification
Essex-Lopresti technique
estrogen
ether
Ethicon suture
ethylene
ethylene oxide
etiology
euploid
Evans procedure
eversion
eversion stress test
evertor
evisceration
evolution
Ewald prosthesis
Ewald scoring system
Ewald total elbow
Ewald and Walker knee implant
Ewing's tumor (sarcoma)
exacerbation
examination
excision

Additional Entries

excoriation
exercise
exfoliation
exoskeleton
exostosectomy
exostosis
exothermic
exotoxin
expander (tissue)
experiment
explant
exploration
exploratory
exposure
exsanguinate
extender
extensile
extension
extensor carpi radialis brevis
(ECRB)
extensor carpi radialis longus
(ECRL)
extensor carpi ulnaris (ECU)
extensor digiti quinti (EDQ)
extensor digitorum brevis
(EDB)
extensor digitorum communis
(EDC)
extensor digitorum longus
(EDL)

extensor hallucis brevis
(EHB)
extensor hallucis longus
(EHL)
extensor hood
extensor indicis proprius
(EIP)
extensor pollicis brevis (EPB)
extensor pollicis longus (EPL)
extensor retinaculum
extensor tendon
external-fixator (fixation)
externalize
extra-articular
extracapsular
extracellular
extract
extraction
extractor
extradural
extramedullary
extraosseous
extravasation
extremity
extrinsic
extrusion
extubate
exuberant
exudate
Eyler procedure

Additional Entries

Additional Entries

F

fabella
fabellofibular ligament
Faber test
facet
facetectomy
facilitative
facioscapulohumeral dystrophy
F.A.C.S. (Fellow of the
   American College of
   Surgeons)
factitious
factor VIII concentrates
factor IX concentrates
factor IX deficiency
Fahey and O'Brian procedure
Fahey approach
Fahrenheit scale
Fairbanks and Sever procedure
false aneurysm
false-negative
false-positive
familial
familial dysautonomia
faradic stimulation
Farmer technique
fascia
fascia lata
fascial

fascial arthroplasty (elbow)
fascialplasty
fascicle
fasciculation
fasciculus
fasciectomy
fascitis
fasciodesis
fasciorraphy
fasciotomy
fast twitch muscle
fat pad sign
fatigue fracture
fatigue strength
fatty tumor
FDA (Food and Drug
   Administration)
febrile
feedback
Feldene
felon
femoral
femoral triangle
femoroiliac
femorotibial
femur
fenestrated
fenestration

Additional Entries

_____
_____
_____
_____
_____
_____
_____
_____

Ferciot technique
Ferguson technique
Ferguson, Thompson, and King
    osteotomy
Ferkel technique
Fernandez osteotomy
ferrous
fetal
fetoprotein
fetus
fiber
fiberoptic
fibril
fibrillation
fibrin
fibrinogen
fibrinoid
fibrinolysin
fibrinolysis
fibroblast
fibrocartilage
fibrocartilaginous
fibrocyte
fibrofatty
fibroma
fibromatosis
fibromyositis
fibroosseous
fibrosarcoma
fibrosis
fibrositis

fibrotic
fibrous
fibrous dysplasia
fibrous union
fibroxanthoma
fibular collateral ligament
fibulocalcaneal
Fielding's classification
figure eight cast
figure eight dressing
figure four position
figure four test
file
Fillauer bar
filum terminale
filum terminale syndrome
finger
    baseball
    clubbed
    mallet
    trigger
    webbed
fingernail
Finkelstein's test
fish mouth amputation
fish mouth suture
Fisher technique
fissure
fistula
five-in-one repair
fixation

Additional Entries

fixator
flaccid
flail
flail joint
Flanagan and Burem graft
flange
flap
    cross-arm
    cross-leg
    free
    island
    local
    pedicle
    rotation
    skin
    sliding
    tubed pedicle
    V-Y
    Z
flare
flatfeet
flatfoot
Flatt prosthesis
flexibility
flexible
flexible pes planus
flexion
flexion contracture
flexion rotation drawer test
flexor
flexor carpi radialis (FCR)

flexor carpi ulnaris (FCU)
flexor digiti minimi
flexor digiti quinti (FDQ)
flexor digitorum brevis (FDB)
flexor digitorum longus (FDL)
flexor digitorum profundus
    (FDP)
flexor digitorum sublimis (FDS)
flexor digitorum superficialis
    (FDS)
flexor hallucis brevis (FHB)
flexor hallucis longus (FHL)
flexor origin
flexor pollicis brevis (FPB)
flexor pollicis longus (FPL)
flexor retinaculum
flexor tendons
flexor zones (hand)
flexorplasty
floating knee
floating ribs
floating thumb
fluorescein
fluoride
fluoroscope
fluoroscopy
fluorosis
fluorouracil (5-FU)
Flynn technique
Flynn, Richards, and Saltzman
    technique

Additional Entries

_____
_____
_____
_____
_____
_____
_____
_____

Foimson biceps tendon repair
fontanelle
foot
    athlete's
    Charcot's
    club
    drop
    flat
    Friedreich's
    Madura
    Morton's
    rocker-bottom
    trench
footdrop
foramen
foramina
foraminotomy
force
forceps
    Adson
    alligator
    bayonet
    mouse-tooth
    thumb
forearm
forefoot
foreign body reaction
forequarter amputation
formaldehyde
formalin
formula

fossa (pl. fossae)
Fournier test
four-flap z-plasty
four-point gait
Fowler technique
Fowles technique
Fox-Blazina procedure
FPB (flexor pollicis brevis)
FPL (flexor pollicis longus)
fracture
    apophyseal
    articular
    avulsion
    Barton's
    basal neck
    bending
    Bennett's
    bimalleolar
    boxer's
    bumper
    bursting
    butterfly
    cleavage
    closed
    Colles'
    comminuted
    complete
    compound
    compression
    condylar
    congenital

Additional Entries

fracture *(continued)*
- depressed
- diacondylar
- direct
- double
- Dupuytren's
- Duverney's
- epiphyseal
- extracapsular
- fatigue
- Galeazzi's
- greenstick
- hangman's
- impacted
- incomplete
- intra-articular
- intracapsular
- intraperiosteal
- intrauterine
- intercondylar
- linear
- longitudinal
- march
- Monteggia's
- Moore's
- multiple
- neoplastic
- oblique
- open
- pathologic
- pertrochanteric

fracture *(continued)*
- pillion
- Pott's
- segmental
- Shepherd's
- simple
- Skillern's
- Smith's
- spiral
- spontaneous
- sprinter's
- stellate
- Stieda's
- subcapital
- stress
- supracondylar
- torsion
- torus
- transcervical
- transcondylar
- transverse
- trimalleolar
- tuft
- Wagstaffe's

fracture-dislocation

fragility

frame
- Balkan
- Bradford
- Foster
- Hibbs'

Additional Entries

frame *(continued)*
    Stryker
    Whitman's
framework
Franke technique
Frankel line
Frankel sign
Frantz and O'Rahilly
    classification
F.R.C.S. (Fellow of the Royal
    College of Surgeons)
free flap
free tendon graft
free-body analysis
Freebody spinal fusion
Freeman resurfacing technique
Freeman-Samuelson prosthesis
Freeman-Swanson prosthesis
freeze-dried bone graft
freeze-drying
Freiberg's disease
Freiberg's infraction
Frejka orthosis (pillow)
French osteotomy (elbow)
fresh frozen plasma (FFP)
friction
Fried technique (clubfoot)
Fried and Hendel transfer
Friedreich's ataxia
frog splint

Frohlich's syndrome
Frohse, arcade of
Froimson procedure
Froment's sign
frontal
frontal plane
fronto occipital
frontoparietal
frontotemporal
frostbite
frozen shoulder
Frykman classification of
    fractures
fulguration
full weight bearing (FWB)
full thickness skin graft (FTSG)
functional fracture brace
fungal
fungicidal
fungus
funicular repair
funiculus
funnel
F.U.O. (fever of undetermined
    origin)
Furacin
furuncle
fusiform
fusimotor
fusion

Additional Entries

G

G-suit
Gaenslen's sign (test)
Gaenslen's procedure
gait
    antalgic
    ataxic
    cerebellar
    Charcot's
    four point
    gluteal
    heel-toe
    hemiplegic
    scissor
    spastic
    steppage
    swing-through
    swing-to
    tabetic
    three-point
    Trendelenburg
    two-point
    waddling
gait training
galactose
galactosemia
Galante's sign
Galeazzi's fracture, sign
Galeazzi's procedure

Gallie needle
Gallie technique
gallium scan
galvanic stimulation
gamekeeper's thumb
gamma globulin
gammopathy
ganglion
ganglionectomy
ganglioneuroma
ganglioside
gangrene
gangrenous
Gant arthrodesis
Gant osteotomy
Garceau approach
Garceau procedure
Garceau Brahms procedure
Garden classification
Gardner approach (shoulder)
Gardner-Wells tongs
gargoylism (Hurler's syndrome)
Garre's osteomyelitis (disease, osteitis)
gas gangrene
gastrocnemius muscle
gastrocsoleus muscle
gastroenteritis

Additional Entries

GAIT (great toe arthroplasty implant technique)
GAIT spacer
gait lock splint (GLS) brace

Gatellier-Chastang approach
  (ankle)
Gaucher's cells, disease
gauge
gauntlet
gauze
gel cast
Gelfoam
Gelpi retractor
gemelli muscle
gene
general anesthesia
general surgery
generic
geneticist
genetics
genicular
geniculate
genitofemoral
genitourinary
gentamicin
gentian violet
genu
    recurvatum
    valgum
    varum
Genucom knee machine
Geometric knee prosthesis
Gerad resurfacing procedure
Gerdy's tubercle
geriatrics

germicidal
germinal matrix
gestation
Getty technique for spinal stenosis
Ghormley technique
Giannestras procedure
giant
giant cell
giant cell tumor
gibbus
Gibney's bandage (strapping)
Gibson approach
gigantism
Gigli saw
Gilbert prosthesis
Gilcreest technique
Giliberty prosthesis
Gill procedure
Gill, Manning, and White fusion
Gill-Stein wrist arthrodesis
Gillies and Millard technique
  (thumb)
Gillies' flap (graft), operation
ginglymus
girdle
Girdlestone procedure
Girdlestone-Taylor tendon
  transfer
Gissane angle
Gissane spike
gland

Additional Entries

glenohumeral
glenoid (fossa)
glenoid labrum
glenoplasty
glioma
globulin
glomus tumor
glucocerebroside
glucocorticoid
glucoprotein
glucosamine
glucose
glucoside
glue
glutaraldehyde
gluteal
gluteus maximus
gluteus medius
gluteus minimus
gluteofemoral
glycine
glycogen
glycolipid
glycolysis
glycoprotein
glycosaminoglycan (GAG)
glycoside
glycosuria
Goldenhaar syndrome
Goldner anterior fusion
Goldner and Clippinger technique

Goldstein spine fusion
Goldthwait's sign
Golgi's complex
gonad
gonadotropin
gonarthritis
gonarthrosis
goniometer
gonococcus
gonorrhea
Gordon technique
Gordon and Bronstrom technique
Gordon and Taylor technique
Gore-Tex graft
Gosselin fracture
Gouffan pin
gouge (pl. gouges)
gout
gouty
gouty arthritis
Gowers' sign
Graber-Duvernay procedure
gracilis muscle
graft
    allograft
    autograft
    bone
    cable
    fascicular
    fat
    free

Additional Entries

Global total shoulder arthroplasty system

graft *(continued)*
    full-thickness
    inlay graft
    Kiel
    nerve
    onlay bone
    pinch
    split-thickness
    Thiersch's
    Wolfe's
    xenograft
Gram's stain
gram-negative
gram-positive
granulation
granulocyte
granuloma
graphite
gravity
Grayson's ligament
grease
grease gun injury
greater multangular
greater saphenous vein
greater sciatic notch
greater trochanter
greater tuberosity
Green procedure
Green and Banks procedure
Green and Grice transfer
Grenlich and Pyle atlas

Grice technique
Grice and Green arthrodesis
grid
grind test
grinding
grip
grip strength
Gritti's amputation
Gritti-Stokes amputation
groin
grommet
groove
Grosse-Kempf nail
growth
growth arrest
growth hormone
growth plate
Guepar knee prosthesis
guide pin
Guillain-Barre' syndrome
guillotine amputation
Guleke-Stookey approach (hip)
gumma
Gunston knee prosthesis
Gurd (Mumford) clavicle resection
Gustilo knee prosthesis
gutter splint
Guttman subtalar arthrodesis
Guyon's amputation
Guyon's canal
gymnastics

Additional Entries

vise-grip

H graft
H & E (hematoxylin and eosin)
   stain
Haas technique
Haddad and Riordan arthrodesis
Haemophilus influenza
Hagie pins
Haglund's deformity
hairline fracture
half-life
Hall drill
Hall technique (facet fusion)
hallucination
hallux
   abductus
   adductus
   dolorosa
   extensus
   flexus
   malleus
   rigidus
   valgus
   varus
halo
halo cast
halo traction
halo wheelchair
halo-femoral traction

halo-pelvic traction
halogen
halothane
hamartoma
hamate bone
hammer
hammertoe
hamstring muscle
hamstrung knee
hand
   benediction
   claw
   cleft
   club
   drop
   Krukenberg's
   lobster-claw
   mirror
   mitten
   opera-glass
   trident
Hand-Schuller-Christian disease
handicap
hanging arm cast
hanging hip procedure
hangman's fracture
hangnail
Hansen's bacillus, disease

Additional Entries

Haid universal bone plate system (UBP system)
Halifax interlaminar clamp system

Hanslik prosthesis (patella)
Hanson-Street nail
haploid
hard corn
hard disc
hardening
hardness
Hare traction splint
Harman approach (tibia)
Harman technique
Harman and Fahey technique
Harrington fusion
Harrington rod
Harris and Beath technique
Harris approach
Harris hip evaluation
Harris line
Harris nail
Harris total hip prosthesis
Hass technique
Hastings procedure
Hauser procedure
haversian canal (space)
Haynes pin
Hawkins sign
head-at-risk signs
healing
health maintenance organization
   (HMO)
heat lamp
heatstroke

Heberden's nodes
hebosteotomy
hebotomy
heel
heel cord
heel pad
heel spur
Heifetz technique (toenail)
height
Heinig procedure
helix
heloma
helotomy
hemangioendothelioma
hemangioma
hemangiopericytoma
hemangiosarcoma
hemarthrosis
hematocrit
hematogenous
hematoma
hematomyelia
hematopoietic
hematoxylin and eosin stain
   (H&E)
hematuria
hemiarthroplasty
hemilaminectomy
hemimelia
hemiparesis
hemipelvectomy

Additional Entries

hemiplegia
hemivertebra
hemochromatosis
hemodialysis
hemodynamic
hemoglobin
hemoglobinopathy
hemoglobinuria
hemogram
hemolysis
hemolytic
hemophilia
hemophiliac
hemorrhage
hemosiderin
hemostasis
hemostat
hemothorax
Henderson approach
Henderson arthrodesis
Henderson graft
Henderson reamer
Henderson technique
Henry approaches
Henry technique
Henry and Geist spinal fusion
Henschke-Mauch SNS knee
heparin
heparinize
hepatitis
Herbert knee prosthesis

Herbert screw
hereditary multiple exostoses
heredity
   autosomal
   sex-linked
   x-linked
Herndon and Heyman procedure
hernia
herniated intervertebral disc
herniation
heroin user
Herold and Torok technique
herpes
herpes zoster
herpesvirus
herpetic whitelow
heterogeneous
heterograft
heterotopic
heterotopic ossification
hex-head screw
hex-head screwdriver
hexachlorophene
Hexelite cast
hexosamine
Hey's amputation (operation)
Hey-Groves technique
Heyman procedure
Heyman, Herndon, and Strong
  technique
Hibbs approach

Additional Entries

Herbert-Whipple bonescrew

Hibbs arthrodesis
Hibbs forceps
Hibbs retractor
Hibbs technique
hibernoma
Hilgenreiner line
Hill-Sachs lesion
hindfoot
hindquarter amputation
hip
hip arthroplasty
hip disarticulation
hip pointer
hip spica
His-Haas procedure
histamine
histiocyte
histiocytoma
histiocytosis
histiocytosis X
histocompatible
histogenesis
histology
Histoplasma
histoplasmosis
Hitchcock procedure
HLA antigen
HNP (herniated nucleus
    pulposus)
Hoagland graft
Hodgen splint (apparatus)

Hodgkin's cells, disease
Hodgson approach (spine
    fusion)
Hoen retractor
Hoffa's disease, operation
Hoffa's fat
Hoffer procedure
Hoffman external fixator
Hoffman-Vital external fixator
Hoffman technique
Hohl classification
Hohmann procedure
Hoke technique
Holt-Oram syndrome
Holt nail
Homan's sign
Homan retractor
homeopathic
homeostasis
homocystinuria
homologous
hood
hook
hormone
hormonotherapy
Horner's syndrome (ptosis)
Horwitz-Adams ankle
    arthrodesis
hospital
hospitalize
hot pack

Additional Entries -

housemaid's knee
Houvanian procedure
Howard technique
Howorth open reduction (hip)
HSS knee prosthesis
Hubbard tank
Huber procedure
Hughston technique
Hughston test
human
humeral
humeroradial
humeroulnar
humerus (pl. humeri)
humpback
Humphry's ligament
Hunter's canal
Hunter rod
Hunter syndrome
Huntington technique
Hurler's syndrome (disease)
hyaline cartilage
hyaluronidase
Hydeltra
hydrarthrosis
hydraulic knee
hydrocephalus
hydrocollator (hot) packs
hydrocortisone
hydrogen peroxide
hydrosyringomyelia

hydrotherapy
hydroxyapatite
25-hydroxycholecalciferol
hydroxylysine
hydroxyproline
hygiene
hygroma
hypalgesia
Hypaque
hyperalgesia
hyperalimentation
hyperbaric oxygen
hypercalcemia
hypercellular
hyperemia
hyperesthesia
hyperextension
hyperflexion
hyperkalemia
hyperkinetic
hyperostosis
hyperparathyroidism
hyperphosphatasia
hyperplasia
hyperreflexia
hypersensitive
hypertelorism
hypertension
hyperthermia
hyperthyroidism
hypertonic

Additional Entries

Hoyer transfer (Phys Ther)

hypertrophic
hypertrophy
hyperuricemia
hypervitaminosis
hypesthesia
hypoactive
hypocalcemia
hypocellular
hypochondriac
hypodactyly
hypoesthesia
hypogastric nerve
hypoglycemia
hypokalemia
hyponychium
hypoparathyroidism
hypophosphatasia
hypophyseal

hypoplasia
hyporeflexia
hypotelorism
hypotension
hypotensive
hypothalamus
hypothenar eminence
hypothenar muscles
hypothermia
hypothermic
hypothesis
hypothyroidism
hypotonic
hypovolemic
hypoxia
hysteresis
hysterical

Additional Entries

iatrogenic
ibuprofen
ICLH arthroplasty
ICU (intensive care unit)
idiopathic
ileus
Ilfield splint
iliac
ilioabdominal
iliococcygeal
iliofemoral
iliofemoroplasty
ilioinguinal
iliolumbar
iliopectineal
iliopsoas
iliosacral
iliotibial
iliotibial band (ITB)
iliotibial tract
ilium
illness
image intensifier
imbricated
immature
immediate fit prosthesis
immobilize
immobilizer

immune
immune globulins
immunity
immunize
immunoassay
immunocomplex
immunocompromised
immunodeficiency
immunodepression
immunoelectrophoresis
immunofluorescence
immunoglobulin
immunology
immunoreaction
immunosuppression
impacted
impactor-extractor
impedance plethysmography
impermeable
impervious
impingement
impingement syndrome
implant
implantation
impotence
impression
impulse
inactivation

Additional Entries

inborn
inbreeding
incasement
inch
incidence
incision
incision and drainage (I & D)
Inclan graft
Inclan-Ober procedure
inclusion cyst
incompatible
incompetent
incomplete
incontinent
incorporation
increment
incubation
incurable
indentation
index finger
Indiana conservative hip
indicator
Indium-111 scan
Indocin
indomethacin
Indong Oh prosthesis
induction
induration
inelastic
infant
infantile cortical hypcrostosis

infarct
infection
infectious
inferolateral
inferomedian
inferoposterior
infestation
infiltrate
infirmary
inflammation
inflammatory
infolding
infra-axillary
infraclavicular
infracostal
infraglenoid
infrapatellar
infrared
infrascapular
infraspinous
infrasternal
infratrochlear
Inglis, Ranawat, and Straub
    approach
Inglis reconstruction
Inglis and Cooper technique
Ingram technique
ingrown toenail
ingrowth
inguinal
INH (isoniazid)

Additional Entries

_____
_____
_____
_____
_____
_____
_____
_____
_____

inheritance
inhibitor
injected
injection
injury
inlay
inlay graft
innervation
innominate artery
innominate bone
innominate osteotomy
inoculate
inoperable
Insall approach (knee)
Insall-Burnstein knee prosthesis
Insall, Burnstein, and Freeman
   total knee
Insall and Hood posterior
   cruciate reconstruction
insert
insertion
insertional activity
insidious
in situ
insoluble
inspection
instep
instrument
instrumentation
integument
interarticular

intercalary
intercarpal
intercondylar
intercondylar notch
intercostal
interdigital neuroma
interdigitate
interbody fusion
interface
interferon
intergluteal
interlocking
intermediate
intermetacarpal
intermetatarsal
intermittent claudication
intermittent traction
intermuscular
intermuscular septum
internal derangement
internal fixation
internal tibial torsion (ITT)
internist
internuclear
interossei muscles
interosseous
interosseous membrane
interpediculate
interphalangeal
interpelviabdominal amputation
interposition

Additional Entries

interpositional arthroplasty
interpubic
interrupted
interscapular
interscapulothoracic amputation
interspace
interspinal
interspinous
interstitial
intertarsal
intertransverse
intertrochanteric
intervertebral
intervertebral discs
intima
intorsion
intra-arachnoid
intra-arterial
intra-articular
intracapsular
intracellular
intractable
intradermal
intradural
intraluminal
intramedullary
intramuscular
intraneural
intraoperative
intraosseous
intrapelvic

intraspinal
intrasynovial
intrathecal
intravascular
intravenous
intravertebral
intrinsic minus deformity
intrinsic muscles
intrinsic plus deformity
intubation
invasive
inversion
inversion stress test
invertor
in vitro
in vivo
involucrum
involuntary
iodine
Iodoform
iodophor
iontophoresis
Iowa hip evaluation
Iowa total hip prosthesis
IPPB (intermittent positive
    pressure breathing)
ipsilateral
iris forceps
iris scissors
irradiation
irreducible

Additional Entries

irregular
irreversible
irrigate
irrigation
irritation
Irwin osteotomy
Irwin technique
ischemia
ischemic
ischial
ischiectomy
ischiococcygeal
ischiofemoral
ischiogluteal bursitis
ischiohebotomy
ischiopubic
ischiorectal
ischiosacral

ischiovertebral
ischium
Ishizuki hinge
island pedicle flaps
isoantibody
isograft
isokinetic
isolation
isometric
isoniazid
Isopaque
isopropyl alcohol
isotonic
isotope
isthmus
I.V. (intravenously)
IVP (intravenous pylegram)

Additional Entries

Additional Entries

J

Jacobson technique (CP)
Jaffe disease
Jahss osteotomy
Jakob reverse pivot shift sign
Jancey nail fold removal
Jamar dynamometer
Janecki-Nelson technique
Jansen's disease
Jansen's test
Japas procedure
JCAH (Joint Commission on
    Hospital Accreditation)
Jebson-Taylor hand function
    test
Jeanne's sign
Jefferson fracture
Jeffery technique
Jendrassik's maneuver
jerk
jerk test
Jewett nail
Jewett orthosis
Johnson technique
Johnson and Spiegel procedure

Johnson-Iowa total hip
Jobst boot
Jobst stocking
joint
joint jack
joint mice
joints of Luschka
Jones and Barnett technique
Jones and Brackett approach
Jones dressing
Jones fracture
Jones technique
Joplin technique
Judet approach (hip)
Judet prosthesis
jugular vein
jump graft
jumper's knee
juvenile
juvenile rheumatoid arthritis
juxtracortical
juxtaephyseal
juxtaposition
juxtaspinal

Additional Entries

Additional Entries

K

Kager's triangle
kanamycin
Kanavel's sign
Kapel technique
Kaplan technique
Kaposi's sarcoma
Kashiwagi technique
Kates forefoot arthroplasty
Kaufer technique
Kauffman test
Keflex
Keflin
Kefzol
Keith needle
Kelikian procedure
Keller procedure
Kellogg Speed spinal fusion
Kelly clamp
Kelly technique
Keloid
Kelvin scale
Ken nail
Kenalog
Kendrick, et al technique (foot)
Kennedy ligament augmenting
  device
Kennedy-Losee modification
  (knee)

keratan sulfate
keratin
keratoma
keratosis
Kerlix dressing
Kermisson elevator
Kernig's sign
Kerr sign
Kerrison rongeur
Kessel and Bonney extension
  osteotomy
Kessler prosthesis
Kessler stitch
Key and Conwell classification
key elevator
Key knee arthodesis
key pinch
Kidner technique
kidney
kidney rest
Kichm, Earle, and DesPrez
  procedure
kiel bone
Kienbock's disease
Kilfoyle classification
kilogram
Kincom tester
kinematics

Additional Entries

_____
_____
_____
_____
_____
_____
_____
_____
_____

kinematic prosthesis
kineplasty
kinesiology
kinesitherapy
kinetic energy
kinetics
Kinetron
King procedure
King and Richards technique
King and Steelquist technique
kink
Kirk technique
Kirkaldy-Willis hip arthrodesis
Kirk's amputation
Kirmisson's operation
Kirner's deformity
Kirschner bow
Kirschner wire
KJ (knee jerk)
Kite corrective cast
Klebsiella
Kleinert technique
Klenzak orthosis
Klinefelter's syndrome
Kling dressing
Klippel-Feil syndrome
Klisic technique
Klumpke's paralysis
Klumpke-Dejerine paralysis, syndrome
knee

knee disarticulation
knee immobilizer
knee jerk (KJ)
knee joint
knee orthoses
knife
Knight-Taylor orthosis
knock-knee
knot
Knott exercises
Knowles pins
knuckle
knuckle pad
Kocher approach
Kocher clamp
Kocher fracture
Kocher manuever
Koch-Mason dressing
Koenig technique (scapula)
Koenig and Schafer approach (ankle)
Kohler's disease
koilonychia
Kramer, Craig, and Noel osteotomy
Kraske's position
Krause-Wolfe graft
Kronner external fixator
Krukenberg's hand (arm)
KT-1000 knee machine
Kudo hinge

Additional Entries

_____
_____
_____
_____
_____
_____
_____
_____
_____

Kuettner technique
Kügelberg-Welander's disease
Kumar, Cowell, and Ramsey
   technique
Kummell's disease (spondylitis)
Küntscher nail (rod)

Kurosaka bone screw
Kutler V-Y flaps
K-wire
kyphoscoliosis
kyphosis
kyphotic

Additional Entries

Additional Entries

LAC (long arm cast)
lacerated
laceration
lacertus fibrosus
Lacey prosthesis
Lachman test
lactic acid
lacuna (pl. lacunae)
lag screw
LAI (Charnley) knee prosthesis
Lamb transfer
Lam modification Jones
    procedure
Lambrinuidi splint
Lambrinuidi procedure
lamella
lamellar bone
lamina (pl. laminae)
laminar air flow
laminated
laminectomy
laminotomy
lance
lancinating
landmark
Landouzy's disease, dystrophy
    (type)

Landouzy-Dejerine dystrophy
    (atrophy, type)
Landsmeer ligaments
Lane bone holding clamp
Lane plates
Lange's operation
Langenbeck's amputation
    elevator
    incision
Langenskiold technique
Langers lines
laparotomy
Lapidus technique
Larmon forefoot arthroplasty
Larrey's amputation (operation)
Larsen's disease
Larsen-Johansson disease
Larson anterior cruciate
    augmentation
Larson hip evaluation
Larson's syndrome
Lasegue's sign
laser
lateral
lateral band
lateralize
latex fixation test

Additional Entries

laciniate ligament

latissimus
latissimus dorsi muscle
lattice
Lauge-Hansen ankle
 classification
Lauenstein's procedure
Laugier's sign
lavage
layer
Leach and Igou osteotomy
lead hand
lead shield
Leadbetter maneuver
Lee graft
Lee needle
Lee technique
leeching
leg
leg length discrepency
Legg-Calve-Perthes disease
 (LCP)
Legg-Perthes disease
Leinbach screw
leiomyoma
Lenart and Kullman technique
L'Episcopo and Zachart
 technique
leprosy
leptomeningitis
Lesch-Nyhan syndrome
lesion

Leslie and Ryan approach
lesser trochanter
lesser tuberosity
Letterer-Siwe disease
leucovorin
leukemia
leukemoid
leukocidin
leukocyte
leukocytosis
leukopenia
Leung's classification
levator
levator scapulae muscle
level
levorotatory
Lewis and Chekofsky femur
 resection
Lichtblau technique (metatarsus)
Liebolt arthrodesis
Liebolt procedure
lidocaine
ligament
ligament augmentation
ligament augmentation device
 (LAD)
ligament of Henry
ligament of Wrisburg
ligamentous
ligamentum flavum

Additional Entries

_____
_____
_____
_____
_____
_____
_____
_____
_____
_____

ligamentum teres
ligate
ligature
light cast
limb
limb girdle
limb girdle dystrophy
limitation
limitation of motion
lincomycin
Lindeman procedure
Linder sign
Lindholm procedure
line
    Blumensat's
    Nelaton's
    Shenton's
    Ullmann's
linea aspera
lineage
linear
liniment
link proteins
linked
Linton and Talbott technique
lipid
lipid reticuloendotheliosis
lipid storage disease
lipofibroma
lipoma
lipomyoma

lipomyxoma
lipoprotein
liposarcoma
lipping
Lipscomb technique
Lipscomb, Henderson, Elkins
    technique
liquefactive
Lisfranc's amputation
Lister tubercle
Little Leaguer's elbow
Little Leaguer's shoulder
Littler procedure
Littler and Cooley technique
Littler and Eaton reconstruction
Littlewood forequarter
    amputation
Liverpool elbow implant
Liverpool knee prosthesis
LLC (long leg cast)
Lloyd-Roberts osteotomy
Lloyd-Roberts and Lettin
    technique
load-bearing
load-sharing
loading
lobster-claw hand
lobster-claw operation
lobster-claw foot
lobulated
local anesthesia

Additional Entries

localized
Localio procedure
locked joint
locomotion
locomotor
LOM (limitation of motion)
London hinge (elbow)
long bone
long thoracic nerve
long tract sign
longevity
longitudinal
loose bodies
Losee procedure (knee)
Losee sign
loosening
lordoscoliosis
lordosis
Lorenz's operation,
 osteotomy
Lorenz's sign
lotion
lumbago
lumbar
lumbarization
lumbodorsal
lumbosacral

lumbrical (pl. lumbrici)
lumen
lunate
lupus erythematosus
Luschka's joints
luxatio erecta
luxation
Lyme arthritis
lymph
lymphadenitis
lymphadenopathy
lymphangiogram
lymphangioma
lymphangiosarcoma
lymphangitis
lymphatic
lymphedema
lymphoblast
lymphocyte
lymphocytosis
lymphoma
lymphosarcoma
lyophilization
lysine
lysis
lysosome
lytic

Additional Entries

_____
_____
_____
_____
_____
_____
_____
_____
_____
_____
_____
_____

MacAusland procedure
MacCarty procedure
maceration
Macewen and Shands osteotomy
MacIntosh knee prosthesis
MacIntosh sign
MacIntosh technique
Macnab and Dall spine fusion
MacNichol and Voutsinas
    classification
macrodactyly
macroglobulinemia
macromolecule
macrophage
macroscopic
Madelung's deformity
Madreporic femoral component
maduromycosis
Madura foot
Maffucci's syndrome
Magilligan technique
magnesium
magnet
magnetic
magnetic resonance imaging
    (MRI)
magnification
Magnuson procedure

Magnuson-Stack procedure
Maisonneuve's amputation,
    fracture
Majestro, Ruda, Frost technique
malacia
maladie
maladjustment
malaise
malalignment
Malawer fibular resection
maldevelopment
male
malformation
Malgaigne's amputation
malignancy
malignant
malignant fibrous histiocytoma
    (MFH)
malignant hyperthermia
malingerer
malingering
malleable
malleolus (pl. malleoli)
mallet finger
mallet toe
malnutrition
malpostition
malpractice

Additional Entries

malrotation
malum coxae senilis
malunion
mandible
maneuver
manipulation
Mankin procedure
Mantelow transfer
Mann technique
Mann and DuVries technique
mannitol
manometer
Manske, McCarroll, and
   Swanson incision
mantle
manual
manubrium
manus
Maquet procedure
Marafioti and Westin rods
marble bones
Marcaine
march fracture
Marfan's syndrome
marfanoid
Marie-Strumpell disease,
   syndrome
Marie-Tooth disease
marker
Marks and Bayne technique
Marlex (graft)

Marmor knee prosthesis
Maroteaux-Lamy syndrome
marrow
Marshall procedure
marsupialization
Martin's bandage
Martin-Gruber communication
Martin screw
Martin technique
masculine
mass
massage
Massie nail
massive osteolysis
MAST (Military Anti Shock
   Trousers)
Master knot of Henry
mastoid
Matchett-Brown prosthesis
material
maternal
Matev procedure
Mathes fascia lata flap
Mathys cementless prosthesis
matrix
mattress (suture)
maturation
mature
Mauck procedure
maxilla
Mayer trapezius transfer

Additional Entries

Mayo bunion repair
Mayo elbow prosthesis
Mayo scissors
Mazas hinge elbow
Mazet knee disarticulation
mcg. (microgram)
McBride bunion repair
McBride prosthesis
McCarroll osteotomy hip
McConnell technique (knee)
McElroy instruments
McElvenny procedure
McFarland tibia grafts
McFarland and Osbourne
   approach
McKee-Farrar hip prosthesis
McKee hinge elbow
McKeever patella prosthesis
McKeever procedure
McLaughlin plate
McLaughlin procedure
McMurray osteotomy
McMurray test
McReynolds procedure
McWhoerter shoulder approach
MD (Doctor of Medicine)
mechanics
mechanoreceptor
medial
medial collateral ligament
   (MCL)

medialis
medialize
median
median nerve
mediastinal
mediastinum
Medicare
medication
medicine
medicolegal
mediolateral
medius
Medrol
medullary
medullary canal
medullary graft
medullary rod (nail)
Mega prosthesis
megakaryocyte
megalodactyly
megavitamin
megavoltage
meiosis
meiotic
melanin
melanoma
melorheostosis
melphalan
membrane
membrancocartilaginous
membranous

Additional Entries

menarche
Mendel's law
Menelaus triple arthrodesis
meninges
meningitis
meningocele
meningomyelitis
meningomyelocele
meniscal
meniscectomy
menisci
meniscosynovial
meniscus
menopause
Mensor and Scheck procedure
menstruation
meperidine hydrochloride
mephenesin
Mephyton
mepivacaine hydrochloride
meprobamate
meralgia paresthetica
Merchant x-r view (knee)
meridian
meromelia
mesenchyma
mesenchymal
mesenchymoma
mesh skin graft
mesoderm
mesomorph

mesoneurium
mesotendon
mesotenon
mesothelium
metabolism
metacarpal
metacarpectomy
metacarpophalangeal
metacarpus
metachromatic
metal
metallergy
metallic
metallosis
metallurgy
metaphase
metaphyseal
metaphyses
metaphysis
metaphysitis
metaplasia
metastasis (pl. metastases)
metastasize
metastatic lesion (tumor)
metatarsal
metatarsalgia
metatarsocuneiform
metatarsophalangeal
metatarsus
    adductocavus
    adductovarus

Additional Entries

metatarsus *(continued)*
    adductus
    brevis
    latus
    primus varus
    varus
methacrylate
methicillin sodium
methocarbamol
method
methotrexate
methylmethacrylate
methylprednisolone
metric
metrizamide
Meyers procedure (hip)
mezlocillin
mg. (milligram)
Michael Reese prosthesis
microanalysis
microanastomosis
microanatomy
microaneurysm
microangiopathy
·microbacteria
microbacterium
microbial
microbicidal
microbiological
microbiology
microcephaly

microcirculation
microcurie
microfilm
micrograph
micromelia
micrometastasis
micromolecular
micro motion
micron
micronize
microorganism
microphotograph
microscope
microscopic
microsome
microsurgery
microvascular
microvilli
midaxilla
midcarpal
midfoot
midget
midsection
midtarsal
migration
Mikhail bone block
Mikulicz angle
Milch procedure
Milk-alkali disease
milkmaids elbow (dislocation)
Milkman's syndrome

Additional Entries

Millender arthroplasty
Millender and Nalebuff wrist
   arthrodesis
Miller/Galante knee
Miller technique
Millesi interfascicular grafts
milliampere
millicurie
milliequivalent
milligram (mg.)
milliliter (ml.)
millimeter (mm.)
millimicron
Milroy's disease (edema)
Milwaukee brace
Milwaukee shoulder
mineral
mineralocorticoid
Minerva cast (jacket)
minimum inhibitory
   concentration (MIC)
Minnesota Multiphasic
   Personality Inventory (MMPI)
mirror hand
Mital elbow release
Mitchell bunionectomy
   (osteotomy)
Mithracin
mithramycin
mitochondria
mitosis

Mittlemeir femoral prosthesis
mobilization
modality
mode
model
modification
Moberg procedure
modulus of elasticity
Moe spinal fusion
Moe plate
mold arthroplasty
molding
moleskin
Molesworth and Campbell
   approach
molybdenum
moment arm
momentum
monarthritis
monarticular
Monckeberg's arteriosclerosis
mongolism
mongoloid
Monk procedure
monoarticular
monochromatic
monoclonal
monoclonal antibody
monocyte
monodactyly
monomer

Additional Entries

mononuclear
monoplegia
monosaccharide
monostotic
monostotic fibrous dysplasia
Monteggia's dislocation, fracture
Montgomery straps
Moore approach
Moore fracture
Moore osteotomy
Moore plate
Moore prosthesis
Morand's foot
morbid
morbidity
morcellation
morgue
moribund
Moro reflex
morphine
morphogenesis
morphology
Morquio's syndrome (disease)
Morquio-Ulrich disease
Morrey total elbow
Morrison toe flap
Morse type taper component
mortality
Morton's toe (disease, foot,
    neuralgia), test
mosaic

mosaicism
Moseley straight line graph
mosquito hemostat
Motrin
movie sign
MS (multiple sclerosis)
mucopolysaccharide
mucopolysaccharidosis
mucoprotein
mucous cyst
Mueller prosthesis
Mueller technique
multifidus
multifocal
multiple myeloma
Munchausen's syndrome
Murphy approach (hip)
muscle
muscle biopsy
muscle pedicle
muscle tone
muscle transfer
muscular
muscular dystrophy (MD)
musculocutaneous
musculocutaneous nerve
musculoskeletal
musculospiral
musculotendinous
Mustard iliopsoas transfer
mutant

Additional Entries

mutation
mutilation
myalgia
myasthenia gravis
myatonia
Mycobacterium infection
Mycobacterium kansassi
Mycobacterium marinum
Mycobacterium tuberculosis
mycosis
myelencephalitis
myelin
myelinated
myelinization
myelinoclasis
myelitis
myelocele
myelocoele
myelodysplasia
myelofibrosis
myelogenesis
myelogram
myelography
myeloma
myelomeningocele
myeloneuritis
myelopathy
myeloplegia
myeloproliferative
myeloschisis
myelosuppressive

myocarditis
myoclonus
myocutaneous
myodynia
myoelectric
myofascial
myofascial release
myofascial treatment
myofascitis
myofibril
myofibrosis
myofibrositis
myofilament
myogenesis
myoglobin
myoglobunuria
myography
myology
myonecrosis
myoneural
myoneuralgia
myopathy
myoplastic
myoplasty
myositis
myositis ossificans
myotome
myotonia
myxadenoma
myxofibroma
myxoma
myxomatous

Additional Entries

Naden-Rieth prosthesis
nafcillin
Naffziger syndrome
Nahai tensor fascia lata flap
nail
nail bed
nail fold
nail-patella syndrome
nail plate
nailing
Nalebuff arthrodesis
Nalfon
nalorphine
nandrolone
Naprosyn
naproxen
narcosis
narcotic
Nassif parascapular flap
natatory ligament
National Association of
    Orthopaedic Nurses (NOAN)
National Association of
    Orthopaedic Technicians
    (NAOT)
nausea
Nautilus equipment
navel
navicular

naviculocapitate
navicular bone
navicular pad
Nebcin
neck-shaft angle
necrosis
necrotic
needle
Neer acromioplasty
Neer classification
Neer prosthesis
negative
Neibauer and Glynn procedure
Neisseria
Neisseria gonorrhea
Nelaton's line
neodymium laser
neomycin
neonatal
neonate
neonatologist
neoplasm
neoplastic
Neoprene
Neosporin
nephrogram
nephrologist
nephropathy
nephrotoxicity

Additional Entries

nerve
nerve block
nerve conduction test
nerve graft
nerve root
nerve sleeve
nervous system
Neufeld nail
neural
neural arch
neuralgia
neurapraxia
neuraxis
neuraxon
neurectomy
neurilemma
neurilemoma
neuritis
neuroanastomosis
neuroanatomy
neuroarthropathy
neuroblastoma
neurocanal
neurocepter
neurocirculatory
neurodynia
neuroectoderm
neurofibril
neurofibroma
neurofibromatosis
neurogenic
neurologic exam

neurologist/neurology
neurolysis
neuroma
neuromotor
neuromuscular
neuromuscular facilitation
neuron
neuropathy
neurorraphy
neurotemesis
neurovascular
neurovascular bundle
neurovascular pedicle
Neviaser procedure
newborn
Newington orthosis
newton
Newton's Law
niacin
Nicola procedure
Nicholas medial compartment
   reconstruction
nickel
Nickel and Perry technique
nicotine
nidus
Niebauer and King open
   reduction (knee)
Niebauer prosthesis
Niemann-Pick disease
night splint
nightstick fracture

Additional Entries

nerve root stretch signs

ninhydrin print test
Nirschl technique (tennis elbow)
nipple
nitrogen
NMR (nuclear magnetic
  resonance) imaging
Nocardia
nociocepter
node
nodular
nodular fasciitis
nodular fibrosis
nodule
Noiles prosthesis
nomenclature
nomogram
nonadherent
nonantigenic
noncemented
noncemented component
nonconductor
nondepolarizer
nondisjunction
noninfectious
noninvasive
nonmyelinated
nonossifying fibroma
non-nucleated
nonspecific
nonsteroidal antiinflamatory
  drug (NSAID)

nonunion
nonviable
non-weight bearing (NWB)
Noonan's syndrome
norepinephrine
Norflex
normal
normal saline
normoblast
normochromic
normotensive
Norwood ITB reconstruction
  (anterior cruciate)
nosocomial
notch
notchplasty
nothing per os (NPO)
notochord
novobiocin
Novocain
Noyes anterior cruciate
  reconstruction
NPO (nothing per os)
Nubain
nuchal
nuclear magnetic resonance
  (NMR) imaging
nuclease
nucleolus
nucleoplasm
nucleoprotein

Additional Entries

Nucleotome Flex II (for removing herniated nucleus pulposus material during spinal surgery)

nucleotide
nucleus
nucleus pulposus
numbness
nurse
nurse practitioner
nursery

nutrient
nutrient artery
nutrition
nutritionist
nylon
nystagmus
nystatin

Additional Entries

O

Ober's operation
Ober's test (sign)
obese
objective
oblique
obliquity
obliteration
obstetric paralysis
obstruction
obturator
occipital
occlude
occlusion
occlusive dressing
occult
occupational therapy (OT)
ochronosis
O'Connor operating scope
O'Donoghue cotton cast
O'Donoghue procedure
O'Donoghue triad
odontoid
off-season conditioning
Ogden classification of fractures
Oh femoral component
ohm
ointment
olecranarthritis

olecranarthropathy
olecranon
olecranon fossa
olecranon impaction syndrome
oligodendroglia
oligomenorrnea
Ollier approach
Ollier graft
Ollier's disease
Ollier-Thiersch graft
Omer technique
Omer and Capen carpectomy
omnipaque
omodynia
omosternum
oncogene
oncogenesis
oncology
Oncovin
oncovirus
onlay graft
ontogeny
onychauxia
onychectomy
onychia
onychocryptosis
onychogenic
onychogryphosis

Additional Entries

onycholysis
onychomycosis
onycho-osteodysplasia
onychopathic
onychosis
onychotomy
Op Site dressing
opaque
open reduction
opening wedge
osteotomy
operable
operate
operating microscope
operating room
operating table
operation
    Adams'
    Adelmann's
    Albee's
    Albee-Delbet
    Albert's
    Anderson's
    Andrew's
    Annandale's
    Barker's
    Barton's
    Barwell's
    Bent's
    Bier's
    Buck's

operation *(continued)*
    Chiene's
    Chopart's
    Codivilla's
    Colonna's
    cosmetic
    Dieffenbach's
    Dupuytren's
    Gant's
    Gill's
    Gillespie's
    Guyon's
    Hey's
    Hibb's
    Hoffa's
    Holme's
    Kirmisson's
    Kocher's
    Konig's
    Larrey's
    Lisfranc's
    Lorenz's
    Macewen's
    Mikulicz's
    Morestin's
    Nelaton's
    Ober's
    Ogston's
    Phemister's
    Pollock's
    Sayre's

Additional Entries

operation *(continued)*
    Syme's
    Teale's
    Thiersch's
    Whitman's
opiate
opisthotonos
Oppenheim's disease
Oppenheim's reflex
opponens
opponensplasty
opportunistic
O.R. (operating room)
O'Rahilly classification
O.R.E.F. (Orthopedic Research and Education Foundation)
Oregon prosthesis
organism
organomegaly
O.R.I.F. (open reduction internal fixation)
O.R.S. (Orthopedic Research Society)
Ortholoc prosthesis
orthopaedic
Orthopaedic Research and Education Foundation (O.R.E.F.)
orthopaedics
orthopedics
orthopedist

orthopod
orthosis
orthotic
orthotist
Orthotron machine
Ortolani sign, test
os calcis
os navicularis
os trigonum
os vesalianum
Osborne and Cotterill technique (elbow)
Osborne approach to hip
Osgood approach
Osgood supracondylar osteotomy of femur
oscillation
Osgood-Schlatter disease
Osler's disease, nodes
Osler-Weber-Rendu disease
osmolarity
Osmond-Clark operation
operation
osmosis
osseotendinous
osseous
ossicle
ossification
ossification centers
ostealgia
ostectomy

Additional Entries

osteitis
   deformans
   fibrosa cystica
   fragilitans
   ossificans
   pubis
ostempyesis
osteoanagenesis
osteoaneurysm
osteoarthritis
osteoarthropathy
osteoarthrosis
osteoarticular
osteoblast
osteoblastoma
osteocampsia
osteocartilaginous
osteochondral
osteochrondral graft
osteochondritis
   deformans juvenilis
   dissecans
   ischiopubica
   juvenilis
   necroticans
osteochondrodysplasia
osteochondrodystrophia
osteochondrofibroma
osteochondrolysis
osteochondroma
osteochondromatosis

osteochondromyxoma
osteochondropathia
osteochondropathy
osteochondrosarcoma
osteochondrosis
osteochondrosis dissecans
osteoclasis
osteoclast
osteoclastic
osteoclastoma
osteocyte
osteodystrophy
osteofibromatosis
osteofluorosis
osteogenesis
osteogenesis imperfecta
osteogenic
osteoid
osteoid osteoma
osteology
osteolysis
osteoma
osteomalacia
osteomyelitis
osteomyelodysplasia
osteon
Osteonics femoral component
osteopath
osteopathy
osteopenia
osteoperiosteal

Additional Entries

osteoperiostitis
osteopetrosis
osteophyte
osteoplasty
osteopoikilosis
osteoporosis
osteoporotic
osteopsathyrosis
osteoradionecrosis
osteorrhaphy
osteosarcoma
osteosclerosis
osteosclerosis fragilis
osteosynthesis
osteotome
osteotomoclasis
osteotomy
Ostrup vascularized rib graft
ototoxic
Otto pelvis

outpatient
outrigger
overcompensation
overdose
overgrafting
overgrowth
overlap
overlay
overriding
over-the-top cruciate repair
Overton spinal fusion
.000 training syndromes
overuse syndromes
overweight
oxacillin sodium
oxadation
oxyxephaly
oxygen
oxyhemoglobin

Additional Entries

Osteotomy types: Austin,
Kelikian "Modified Z", modified Mau,
rotational Scarf, and Scarf.

Additional Entries

P

P.A. (physician assistant)
pachyonychia
Pacinian corpuscles
packing
packs (hot, cold)
pad
Padgett's dermatome
Page procedure
Paget's disease
pagetoid
pain
    heterotopic
    lancinating
    phantom limb
    referred
    rest
    root
    shooting
paint gun injury
Palacos cement
palliate
palliative
pallor
palm
palmar
palmar fascia
palmar fasciectomy
palmar fasciotomy

palmar fibromatosis
palmaris longus muscle
palmaris longus tendon
palpable
palpation
palsy
panarthritis
Pancoast's tumor
pancytopenia
pandemic
panhypopituitarism
Panner's disease
pannus
pantalar fusion
Pantopaque
papain
Papineau sequestrectomy and
    curettage
papaverine
paracentesis
paraffin
paraffin bath
Parafon Forte
parahormone
parallel bars
paralysis
paralytic
paramedian

Additional Entries

_____
_____
_____
_____
_____
_____
_____
_____
_____

parameniscus
parameter
paraplegic
parapodium orthosis
pararectal
parasacral
parasagittal plane
parasternal
parasympathetic
paratenon
parathormone
parathyroid
parathyroidectomy
paravertebral
paraxial
parenchyma
parenchymal
parenteral
paresis
paresthesia
Parham band
parhormone
parietal
Parkinson's disease
parkinsonism
paronychia
parosteal
paroxysmal
Parrish procedure
parrot-beak meniscus tear
pars defect

pars interarticularis
partial meniscectomy
partial weight-bearing (PWB)
passive joint movement
passive range of motion
Pasteurella
patella
patella alta
patella baja
patellar compression syndrome
petellar index
patellar tendon
patellar tracking
patellectomy
patellofemoral
patelloplasty
patent
paternal
Paterson procedure
    (pseudarthrosis of tibia)
pathogenesis
pathognomonic
pathologic fracture
pathologist
pathology
pathophysiology
patient
Patrick's test
Pauwels angle
Pauwels fracture
Pauwels osteotomy

Additional Entries

Pauwels Y osteotomy
Pavlik harness
PCA hip, knee
PCL (posterior cuciate ligament)
Peabody classification of foot
    and ankle paralysis
Peabody tibialis tendon transfer
Peacock transposition of index
    ray
Pearson attachment
pectoral
pectoralgia
pectoralis
pectoralis major muscle
pectoralis minor muscle
pectus carinatum
pectus excavatum
pedal
pedal pulse
pediatrician
pediatrics
pedicle
pedigree
pedograph
PEEP (positive end-expiratory
    pressure)
Peet technique for leg
    constrictures
peg
peg graft
pellagra

Pellegrini's disease
Pellegrini-Stieda disease
Pellizzi's syndrome
pelvic
pelvic femoral angle
pelvic obliquity
pelvic ring fractures
pelvic sling
pelvic tilt
pelvic traction
pelvifemoral
pelviotomy
pelvirectal
pelvis
pelvisacral
pelvisacrum
penetrating
penicillamine
penicillin
penicillinase
penicillin-fast
pennate muscles
Penrose drain
pentadactyl
pentazocine
peptide
Peptostreptococcus
Percocet
Percodan
percussion
percutaneous

Additional Entries

percutaneous pinning
perforation
perforator
performance
perfuse
perfusion
periarteritis
periarthritis
periarticular
periarticular fibrositis
peribursal
pericapsular
perichondrial
perichondritis
perichondrium
perichondroma
pericyte, Zimmerman's
peridural
perimysium
perineum
perineurial fibrosis
perineurium
perionychia
perionychium
perioperative
periosteal
periosteal callus
periosteal chondroma
periosteal chondrosarcoma
periosteal desmoid
periosteal elevator

periostitis
periosteodema
periosteomyelitis
periosteotomy
periosteum
periostitis
periostosis
peripatellar
peripheral
peripheral vascular disease
peripheroceptor
peritendinitis
peritenon
peritoneum
perivascularity
perivertebral
Perkins vertical reference line
permeate
peroneal
peroneotibial
peroneus brevis muscle
peroneus brevis tendon
peroneus longus muscle
peroneus longus tendon
peroneus tertius muscle
peroxide
per primam
Perry procedure
Perry, O'Brien, and Hodgson
    technique
Perthes disease

Additional Entries

pes
    abductus
    adductus
    anserinus
    cavus
    congential convex valgus
    equinovalgus
    equinovarus
    planovalgus
    planus
    pronatus
    supinatus
    valgus
    varus
pes anserine
pes anserine bursitis
petechiae
Petrie spica cast
petrolatum
phagocyte
phagocytosis
phalangeal
phalangectomy
phalanges
phalangette
phalangization
phalanx (pl. phalanges)
Phalen test
Phalen-Miller procedure
phantom limb
phantom pain

pharmaceutical
pharmacist
pharmacology
pharmacy
phase
Pheasant technique
Phelps brace
Phelps gracilis test
Phelps-Baker gracilis test
Phemister approach
Phemister graft
phenacetin
Phenergan
phenobarbital
phenol
phenol nerve block
phenolization
phenothiazine
phenotype
phenylalanine
phenylbutazone
phenylketonuria
Pierrot and Murphy technique
Phillips screw
pHisoHex
phlebectasia
phlebectomy
phlebitis
phlebogram
phebothrombosis
phocomelia

Additional Entries

Phoenix total hip prosthesis
phonarteriogram
phonophoresis
phosphatase
    acid p.
    alkaline p.
    serum p.
    phosphate
    calcium p.
phosphaturia
phospholecithinase
phospholipid
phosphonate
phosphoproteins
phosphorus
phosphorylase
phosphorylation
photomicrograph
photon
physeal
physiatrics
physiatrist
physical exam
physical fitness
Physical Medicine and
    Rehabilitation (PM & R)
physical therapy (PT)
physician
physician assistant (PA)
physiology
physiotherapist

physiotherapy
physis
physostigmine
pia-arachnoid
pia mater
Piedmont fracture
piezoelectric effect
pigmentation
pigmented
pigmented villonodular synovitis
  (PVS)
pillar
pillow splint, triangular
pilonidal cyst
pilonidal sinus
pimple
pin
pin tract
pin tract infection
pin tract sinus
pinch
pinched nerve
pinch graft
PIP (proximal interphalangeal)
  joint
Piperacillin
piriform sinus
piriformis muscle
piriformis syndrome
Pirogoff's amputation
Pirogoff's angle

Additional Entries

piroxicam
pisiform
pitting
pitting edema
Pittsburgh triangular frame
pituitary gland
pituitary rongeur
pivot shift test
PKU (phenylketonuria)
placebo
placenta
plafond fracture
plagiocephaly
plane
    axial p.
    coronal p.
    horizontal p.
    frontal p.
    median p.
    midsagittal p.
    sagittal p.
    transverse p.
    vertical p.
planigram
planoconcave
planoconvex
plantar
plantar aponeurosis
plantar fascia
plantar flexion
plantar wart

plantaris muscle
plantaris tendon
plantigrade
plaque
Plaquenil
plasma
plasmablast
plasmacyte
plasmacytosis
plaster
plaster of Paris
plastic
plasticity
Plastizote
plate
    A.O.
    bone
    compression
    Eggers'
    Lane
    malleable
    Moe
    Sherman
    supracondylar
    T
    Y
plate of Driessen
plateau
platelet
plating
platform system (ankle)

Additional Entries

platybasia
platycephalic
platyonychia
platypodia
platysma
platyspondylisis
pledget
pleomorphic
plethysmograph
plexiform
plexus
plica (pl. plicae)
plicae
plicate
plication
pliers
pluripotential
PM & R (Physical Medicine and Rehabilitation)
PMMA (polymethylmethacrylate)
pneumarthrogram
pneumarthrography
pneumarthrosis
pneumatic
pneumatic tourniquet
Pneumocycstis
pneumoencephalogram
pneumohemothorax
pneumomediastinum
pneumonia

pneumonitis
pneumothorax
P.O. (by mouth)
podagra
podiatrist
podiatry
podogram
pointer (hip)
Poland classification of fractures
Poland syndrome
polarity
polarization
Polaroid film (X-R)
pole
polio
poliomyelitis
poliomyelopathy
poliovirus
pollicization
polyalgesia
polyarteritis
polyarteritis nodosa
polyarthritis
polycentric
polycentric knee prosthesis
polyclinic
polyclonal
polydactyly
polyethylene
polymer
polymerization

Additional Entries

polymetacarpia
polymetatarsia
polymethylmethacrylate
  (PMMA)
polymicrobial
polymorphism
polymyalgia
polymyositis
polymyxin B. sulfate
polyneuritis
polyneuropathy
polynuclear
polyostotic
polypeptide
polyperiostitis
polyphalangia
polyplegia
polypropylene
polysaccharide
polysyndactyly
polyurethane
polyvinyl
Pontocaine
popliteal
popliteal cyst
popliteus muscle
popliteus syndrome
porcelain
porous
porous ingrowth
portal

Porter, Richardson, and Vainio
  elbow synovectomy
position
positive
postacetabular
postaxial
postbrachial
postclavicular
postcondylar
postcubital
posterior
posterior drawer test
posterior interosseous nerve
posterior longitudinal ligament
posterior sag sign
posterior triangle
posteroanterior
posteroinferior
posterolateral
posteromedial
posteromedian
posterosuperior
postganglionic
postglenoid
postirradiation
postmenopausal
post mortem
postnatal
postop
postoperative
post-polio syndrome

Additional Entries

postradiation
postsacral
postscapular
postsynaptic
post-tarsal
post-tibial
post-traumatic
postural
posture
potassium
potential
Potenza arthrodesis
Pott's disease
Pott fracture (ankle)
Pott tibial osteotomy
Potter knee arthrodesis
Pott's paraplegia
pouch
Poupart inguinal ligament
povidone
povidone-iodine
powder
P.P.D. (purified protein derivative)
practitioner
preanesthetic
preaxial
precancerous
preclinical
precollagenous
precursor
predisposing

predisposition
prednisilone
prednisone
preganglionic
pregnancy
pregnant
prehallux
prehensile
prehension
Preiser's disease
preleukemia
premalignant
Premarin
premature
premedication
premenstrual
premenstrual syndrome (PMS)
prenatal
preop
preoperative
preparticipation exam
prepatellar
prepatellar bursitis
preprosthetic
PREs (Progressive Resistance
    Exercises)
presacral
prescapular
prescription
preservative
prespondylolisthesis

Additional Entries

_____
_____
_____
_____
_____
_____
_____
_____
_____

press-fit prosthesis
pressure
    arterial p.
    blood p.
    capillary p.
    central venous p. (CVP)
    cerebrospinal p.
    diastolic p.
    hydrostatic p.
    intra-abdominal p.
    intracranial p.
    intrathecal p.
    negative p.
    perfusion p.
    positive p.
    positive end-expiratory
      pressure (PEEP)
    pulse p.
    systolic p.
    venous p.
presynaptic
pretarsal
pretibial
prevalence
preventive
prevertebral
Pridie-Koutsogiannis technique
primary
primary nerve repair
primary skin closure
primary tendon suture

prime mover (muscle)
primordial
Pritchard-Walker hinge (elbow)
p.r.n.
proatlas
proband
probe
probenecid
procaine
procarbazine
procedure
process
prochlorperazine
procollagen
procollangenase
prodrome
professional
Professional Standards Review
    Organization (PSRO)
profile
profundus
profundus tendon
prognosis
progressive
progressive resistance exercise
    (PREs)
prolapse
proliferation
proline
prominence
pronation

Additional Entries

_____
_____
_____
_____
_____
_____
_____
_____
_____

pronatoflexor
pronator
pronator quadratus muscle
pronator teres muscle
prone
prone rectus test
prong
prophase
prophylactic
prophylactic antibiotics
prophylaxis
Proplast
propoxyphene
proprioception
proprioceptor
propriospinal
prostaglandin
prostate
Protasul femoral prosthesis
protective pads
prothesis
prosthetic
prosthetist
protease
protein
proteinase
proteoglycan
proteolytic
Proteus
prothrombin
prothrombin time (PT)

protocol
protoplasm
prototype
protovertebra
protraction
protractor
protrusio
protrusio acetabuli
protrusion
protuberance
provertebra
proximal
proximal focal femoral
  deficiency (PFFD)
proximal interphalangeal (PIP)
  joint
pseudarthrosis
pseudocyst
pseudoepiphysis
pseudofracture
pseudoganglion
pseudogout
pseudohypertrophic
pseudohypertrophic dystrophy
pseudohypoparathyroidism
pseudohypophosphatasia
pseudoluxation
pseudomeningocele
Pseudomonas
pseudoneuroma
pseudoparalysis

Additional Entries

pseudotabes
psoas muscle
psoas tendon
psoriasis
psoriatic arthritis
PSRO (Professional Standards
 Review Organization)
psychogenic
psychologic
psychologic testing
psychomotor skills
PTT (partial thromboplastin
 time)
puberty
pubiotomy
pubis
pubic ramus
Puddu reconstuction
Pugh nail
pull-out suture (wire)
pull-ups
pulley exercises
pulmonary
pulmonary emboli
pulmorary function test
pulp
pulsatile
pulsation
pulse
Pulvertaft suture
pump bump

punch
punched-out
punctate
puncture
purine
Purkinje's cells
Purkinje's fibers
purpura
purulent
pus
pustule
putrefy
Putti and Abbott approach
Putti approach
Putti arthrodesis
Putti technique
Putti-Platt operation
Putti-Scaglietti procedure
putty
pyarthrosis
pyelogram
pyemia
pygmy
pyknodysostosis
pylon
pyogenic
pyogenic granuloma
pyrexia
pyridoxine
pyruvate

Additional Entries

_____

_____

_____

_____

_____

_____

_____

_____

Additional Entries

Q

Q angle (knee)
q.d. (every day)
q.i.d. (four times a day)
quad atrophy
quadrant
quadratus muscle
quadratus femoris muscle
quadratus lumborum muscle
quadratus plantaris muscle
quadriceps muscle

quadricepsplasty
quadrilateral
quadriplegia
quadriplegic
qualitative
quantitative
quarter
quarterback
Queckenstedt sign
quinine

Additional Entries

Additional Entries

rabies
rachialgia
rachiopathy
rachiotomyrachis
rachisagra
rachischisis
rachitic
rachitis
rachitome
racquet
rad
radial
radial clubhand
radial collateral ligament
radial deviation
radial drift
radial head
radial tunnel
radial tunnel syndrome
radiate
radiation
radiation therapy
radical
radicular
radiculectomy
radiculitis
radiculoneuritis
radiculopathy

radioactivity
radiocarpal
radiodensity
radiodermatitis
radiodigital
radiograph
radiography
radiohumeral
radioimmunity
radioimmunoassay
radioisotope
radioisotopic scan
radiologist
radiology
radiolucent
radionecrosis
radioneuritis
radionuclide
radiopacity
radiopaque
radioresistance
radiosensitive
radiotherapist
radiotherapy
radioulnar
radium
radius
Radley-Liebig-Brown technique

Additional Entries

ragocyte
ramus
Ranawat, Defiore and Straub
    technique
range of motion (ROM)
rarefaction
Raynaud's disease (gangrene)
Rapp technique (serratus anterior)
ray amputation
Raynaud's phenomenon
reamer
reamputation
rearfoot
reattachment
rebound
recalcification
receptor
recession
recessive
reciprocation
Recklinghausen's disease
recondition exercises
reconstitution
reconstruction
recruitment
rectal
rectilinear
rectum
rectus muscles
recumbent
recuperation

recurrent
recurvatum
recurvatum test
redislocation
reduce
reduced
reducible
redundant
reduplication
re-education
Reese dermatome
referred pain
reflection
reflex
    abdominal
    Achilles tendon
    ankle
    Babinski's
    biceps
    cremasteric
    grasp
    grasping
    Hoffmann's
    knee jerk (quadriceps jerk)
    rooting
    startle (Moro's)
    stepping
    triceps
reflex sympathetic dystrophy
    (RSD)
refractory
refracture

Additional Entries

Refsum's syndrome
regeneration
regimen
regional
regional anesthetic (block)
registered occupational therapist
regression
rehabilitation
Reichenheim technique (elbow)
Reid and Baker procedure (ulna)
reimplantation
reinfection
reinforcement
reinnervation
Reiter's syndrome
rejection
relapse
relaxant
release
relieve
remineralization
remission
remnant
Rendu-Osler-Weber disease
repair
replantation
replication
repolarization
reposition
reproduction
resection

resection-arthrodesis
reserpine
resident
resin
resistance
resorb
respirator
respiratory
restoration
rest pain
resultant force
resuscitation
resurfacing
retainer
retention
reticuloendothelial
retinaculum
reticulum cell sarcoma
retinacula, medial and lateral
retraction
retractor
retrocalcaneobursitis
retrograde
retropatellar
retroperitoneal
retroperitoneum
retrosternal
retroversion
revascularization
Reverdin osteotomy
Reverdin skin graft

Additional Entries

Regnauld-type degeneration

Reverdin-Green procedure
reverse last shoes
reversible
revision
RF (rheumatoid factor)
rhabdomyosarcoma
rhachotomy
rheumatism
rheumatoid
rheumatoid arthritis (RA)
rheumatoid factor (RF)
rheumatologist
rheumatology
Rh factor
rhythmn (Circadian)
rhizomelic
rhizotomy
rhomboid major muscle
rhomboid minor muscle
rib
rib belt
rib graft
ribosome
rib-vertebral angle
rice bodies
Richards, Saltzman, and Flynn
   technique
Riche-Cannieu anastomosis
rickets
ridge
right-angled retractor

right-angled sutures
rigid fixation
rigid orthosis
rigidity
rim
ring avulsion injury
ring epiphyses
Ring knee prosthesis
Ring total hip prosthesis
Ringer's lactate
Riordan procedure
risk factors
Riseborough and Radin
   classification (humeral
   fractures)
Risser localizer cast
Roaf approach
Robert Brigham prosthesis
Robert Jones bandage
Roberts approach
Robinson and Riley cervical
   arthrodesis
Robinson and Southwick fusion
Robinson procedure
Rocephin
rocker-bottom foot
Rockwood classification (A-C
   joint)
Rockwood and Green technique
roentgenogram
Roger Anderson external fixator

Additional Entries

Rogozinski spinal rofourter

Rolando fracture
roll stitch
ROM (range of motion)
   exercises
rongeur
Rood proprioceptive
   neuromusclar facilitation
   (PNF)
Roos transaxillary approach
Rose procedure
rotary subluxation
rotation
rotational instability
rotator cuff

rouleaux formation
Roux-Goldthwait procedure
Rowe posterior approach
   (shoulder)
Royle-Thompson FDS transfer
RNA
rudimentary
Ruiz-Moro procedure
running shoe
rupture
Russe bone graft
Russell-Taylor interlocking nail
Russell's traction
Ryerson triple arthrodesis

Additional Entries

Additional Entries

Saba's classification (shoulder muscles)
saber-cut incision
sac
sacral
sacral agenesis
sacral plexus
sacralgia
sacralization
sacrectomy
sacrococcygeal
sacrocoxalgia
sacrodynia
sacroiliac
sacroiliac belt
sacroiliac joint
sacroilitis
sacrolistheis
sacrolumbar
sacroperineal
sacrospinal
sacrospinous ligament
sacrotuberous ligament
sacrovertebral
sacrovertebral angle
sacrum
safety pin orthosis
Sage rod

Sage technique
Sage and Clark cheilectomy
Sage and Salvatore classifiction (A-C joint injuries)
sagittal
Saha procedure
Sakellarides technique (forearm contracture)
salicylate
saline
saline dressing
salmonella
salsalate
Salter fracture
Salter-Harris fracture
Salter innominate osteotomy
Saltzman, Flynn, and Richards technique
salvage
salve
Samilson osteotomy (calcaneus)
Sanfilippo syndrome
saphenous
saphenous nerve
saphenous vein
sarcoblast
sarcoidosis
sarcolemma

Additional Entries

_____
_____
_____
_____
_____
_____
_____
_____
_____

sarcoma
sarcomere
sarcoplasm
Sarmiento cast
Sarmiento osteotomy
saucerization
Scaglietti procedure
scalene
scalenotomy
scalenus anticus muscle
scalenus anticus syndrome
scalenus medius muscle
scalenus posticus muscle
scalpel
scan
scanner
scaphoid
scapula
scapulectomy
scapulopexy
scapuloclavicular
scapulohumeral
scar
Schaeffer orthosis
Schanz osteotomy
Schanz screws
Schauwecker compression
  wiring (patella)
Scheck and Mensor hanging hip
  operation
Schede osteotomy

Scheier hinge (elbow)
Scheuermann's disease
Schmorl's disease
Schmorl's nodule
Schneider arthrodesis
Schneider nail (rod)
Schneider technique
Schnute's wedge resection
  (osteitis pubis)
Schuller-Christian disease
Schwann's cell
Schwann tumor
Schwannoma
Schwartz and Baumgard
  technique (tennis elbow)
sciatic
sciatic notch
sciatica
scintigram (scintiscan)
scissors
sclera
scleroderma
sclerosing osteomyelitis of Garre
sclerosis
scoliokyphosis
scoliosis
scoliotic
Scott glenoplasty
Scottish Rite orthosis
Scottish Rite procedure
scout film

Additional Entries

_____
_____
_____
_____
_____
_____
_____
_____
_____

screw home mechanism
(knee)
Scuder technique
scurvy
seat belt injury
sebaceous cyst
secondary closure
secondary ossification center
second-degree burn
second-degree sprain
second generation (antibiotic)
section
sedation
Seddon arthrodesis
Seddon costotransversectomy
sediment
sedimentation rate
segment
segmental fracture
segmental graft
segmental innervation
Seinsheimer classification
(subtrochanteric fractures)
seizures
self-compressing plate
self-induced injury
self-limited
self-tapping bone screw
sella turcica
semiconstrained prosthesis
semi-Fowler position

semiinvasive electrical
stimulation systems
semilunar
semimembranous
semimembranosus muscle
semimembranosus tendon
semitendinosus muscle
semitendinosus tendon
semitubular plate
senile
sensibility
sensitivity
sensitization
sensorimuscular
sensory
sensory deficit
sensory evoked potentials
(SSEP)
sepsis
septic
septic arthritis
septicemia
septum
sequestrum
sequestrectomy
serial wedged cast
series
serious
serology
seroma
seronegative

Additional Entries

seropositive
serosanguineous
serotonin
serotype
serous
serrated
Serratia
serratus anterior muscle
serum
serum sickness
sesamoid
sesamoiditis
sessile
sessile osteochondroma
Sevastano knee prosthesis
Sever operation
severed
Sever's disease
sex-linked
shaft
Schanz dressing
sharp
Sharpey's fibers
Sharrard iliopsoas transfer
shear force
shear modulus
shear strain
shear stress
sheath
Sheehan knee prosthesis
shelf

shelf procedure
Shenton's line (arch)
Shepherd's fracture
Sherk and Probst technique
Sherman bone plates
Shiers knee prosthesis
shin
shin splints
shingles
shock
shock absorption
shoe
shoe insert
shoe lift
shoe wedge
short arc exercises
short arm cast (SAC)
short leg cast (SLC)
short leg walking cast (SLWC)
short wave diathermy
shoulder
shoulder impingement syndrome
SI (sacroiliac) joint
sibling
sickle cell anemia
sickle cell disease
sideswipe fracture
Siegel technique
Siffert, Forster, Nachamie
    technique
Silastic

Additional Entries

_____
_____
_____
_____
_____
_____
_____
_____
_____

Silesian bandage
Silfverskiold procedure
silicone rods
Silvadene
Silver procedure
silver-fork deformity
Silverman's needle
Simmonds and Menelaus
    technique
Simmons osteotomes and chisels
Simmons technique
Simplex cement
Sinding-Larsen-Johansson
    disease
Singh index
sinogram
sintered
sinus
sinus tarsi
sinus tarsi syndrome
sinus tract
sit-ups
Sivash prosthesis
Sjogren's syndrome (disease)
skeletal
skeletal muscle
skeleton
skewfoot
Skillern's fracture
skin creases
skin graft

skin traction
Skoog technique
skull
SLAC (Scapho-Lunate
    Advanced Collapse)
SLE (systemic lupus
    erthymatosus)
slide
sliding graft
sliding nail
sling
sling-and-swathe bandage
slipped capital femoral epiphysis
slit
slit lamp
Slocum anterior rotary drawer
    test
Slocum technique
slope
slough
slow-twitch fibers (white)
Smillie nail
Smith fracture
Smith prosthesis
Smith technique
Smith and Robinson anterior
    approach
Smith's dislocation, fracture
Smith-Peterson arthrodesis
Smith-Petersen cup
Smith-Petersen nail

Additional Entries

snapping tendons
snare
snuffbox
soccer-style kicker
socket
sodium
Sofield osteotomy
soft disc
softening
soft tissue
sole
solid
solid ankle cushioned heel
  (SACH)
solitary
solitary myeloma
soluble
Solu-Cortef
solution
solvent
Soma
Soma compound
somatic
somatoplasm
somatotype
Somerville open reduction (hip)
sonogram
sore
Soto-Hall patellectomy
Souter hinge (elbow)
Southwick osteotomy

Southwick and Robinson
  approach
space shoes
spacer
spasm
spastic
spasticity
spatula
spearing (football)
specialist
specimen
spectinomycin
Spectron femoral component
Speed osteotomy
Speed and Boyd open reduction
sphenoid
spherical
sphincter
sphingolipid
sphingolipidosis
sphingolipodystrophy
sphingomyelin
sphingomyelinosis
spica bandage
spica cast
spicule
Spier elbow arthrodesis
spike
spina bifida
spina bifida occulta
spinal

Additional Entries

_____
_____
_____
_____
_____
_____
_____
_____
_____

spinal accessory nerve
spinal block
spinal board
spinal canal
spinal cord
spinal fusion
spinal nerve
spinal process
spinal puncture
spinal stenosis
spinalis muscle
spindle
spine
spinocerebellar
spinothalamic tract
Spira procedure
spiral
spiral fracture
spiral groove
splayfoot
spleen
splenectomy
splenius muscle
splenomegaly
splint
splinter
split Russell traction
split thickness skin graft (STSG)
splitting
spondylalgia
spondylarthritis

spondyloarthracae
Spondyloepiphyseal dysplasia
spondyloexarthrosis
spondylitis
spondylodesis
spondylodynia
spondylolisthesis
spondylolisthetic
spondylolysis
spondylosyndesis
spondylotomy
spondylopathy
spondyloschisis
sponge
Sponsel osteotomy
sports medicine
sports psychologist
spondylosis
spongiosa
spoon nail
sporotrichosis
sprain
spreader
spreader bar
Sprengel's deformity
spring ligament
spring swivel thumb
sprinter's fracture
spur
Spurling test
SQ (subcutaneous)

Additional Entries

_____
_____
_____
_____
_____
_____
_____
_____
_____

squatting
squinting patellae
SSEP (somatosensory evoked
    potentials)
stab
stability
stable
Stack splint
Stagnaara wake-up test
Staheli shelf operation
stainless steel
stalk
Stamm arthrodesis
standard deviation
standing frame orthrosis
Stanisavljevic technique
Stanmore total hip
staphylococcal
Staphylococcus aureus
Staphylococcus epidermidis
staple gun
stapler
stasis
stasis ulcer
static
station
stationary bicycle
statistics
stature
Steichen technique (toe)
Steindler technique

Steinmann pin
stellate
stellate block
stellate ganglion block
stem
Stener and Gunterberg sacrum
    resection
stenosed
stenosing tenosynovitis
stenosis
stent
stent dressing
step-cut lenghtening
step-up exercises
Stephenson and Donovan
    transfer
stereognosis
sterile
sterile field
sterilization
sterilizer
sternal
sternalgia
Sternberg-Reed cells
sternoclavicular
sternocleidomastoid muscle
sternocostal
sternotomy
sternum
steroid
stethoscope

Additional Entries

Steward technique
Steward and Harley ankle
   arthrodesis
Stewart technique
Stieda's disease
Stieda's fracture
stiffness
stiffness coefficient
Stiles-Bunnell transfer
Still's disease
Stimson maneuver
stimulator
stimulus
stinger injury
stippled epiphysis
stippling
stirrup
stitch
stockinette
Stone procedure
Stone staple
Stone hip arthrodesis
straight last shoes
straight leg raising (SLR) test
straight stem femoral
   components
straight-stemmed
strain
strain energy
strait
strap

strapping
stratification
Strauab technique (ulna)
strawberry hemangioma
Strayer procedure
Street diamond-shaped nail
Street and Stevens humeral
   replacement
Streeter's dysplasia
strength
strength testing
strength training
streptococcus
streptokinase
streptolysin
streptomycin
stress
stress fracture
stress roentgenogram
stress-strain curve
stress test
stretch
stretch reflex
stretch exercises
stretcher
striated
Strickland tendon repair
stricture
stride
stride length
strike

Additional Entries

stripper
stroke
stroma
structure
Strumpell-Marie disease
strut graft
Stryker dermatome
Stryker saw, equipment
stump
stump shrinker
stump sock
stylet
styloid
styoidectomy
styloid process
subacromial
subacute
subastraglar
subarachnoid
subcapital fracture
subchondral
subchondral bone
subclavian
subclavian artery
subclavian steal syndrome
subclavian vein
subclavicular
subclinical
subcostal
subcutaneous
subcuticular

subdeltoid
subdural
subjective
subluxation
subperiosteal
sub-Q (SQ)
subscapular
subscapularis muscle
subscapularis tendon
subspecialty
substance
substitution
subtalar
subtraction
subungual
subungual exostosis
subungual hematoma
succinylcholine
suction drain
Sudeck's atrophy
sugar tong cast
sugar tong splint
Sugioka transtrochanteric
    osteotomy
sulcus
sulcus angle
sulfamethazine
sulfinpyrazone
sulfonamide
sulindac
sunrise view

Additional Entries

sunset view
superficial
superinfection
superior
supernatant
supernumerary
superolateral
superomedial
superstructure
supervoltage
supinate
supination
supinator muscle
supine
Suppan procedure
support
support stockings
suppository
suppressant
suppurative
supraclavicular
supracondylar
supraglenoid
supramalleolar
suprapatellar
suprapatellar plica
suprapatellar pouch
suprapubic
suprascapular
supraspinal
supraspinatus muscle

supraspinatus tendon
supraspinous
suprasternal
suprasternal notch
supratrochlear
surface
surface electrodes
surfactant
surgeon
surgery
surgibone
surgical
surgical assistant
surgical neck fracture
surgical shoe
Surgicel
susceptible
suspended traction
suspension
suspensory
sustentacular
sustentaculum
Sutherland hamstring transfer
Sutherland and Greenfield
    osteotomy
suture
Swanson classification
    (congenital skeletal limb
    deficiency)
Swanson Silastic prosthesis
swan neck deformity

Additional Entries

swayback
sweat test
Swedish knee cage
swelling
swimmer's knee
swing phase (gait)
swollen
symbrachydactyly
Syme's amputation, operation
symmetrical
sympathectomy
sympathetic nervous system
sympathomimetic
symphalangia
symphalangism
symphysis pubis
symptom
symptom complex
synapse
synarthrosis
synchondrosis
synchronous
syncope
syncytium
syndactyly
syndesmosis
syndrome
synergist

synergy
synostosis
synovectomy
synovia
synovial
synovial chondromatosis
synovial cyst
synovial fluid
synovial joint
synovial membrane
synovial osteochondromatosis
synovial plicae
synoviochondromatosis
synoviogram
synovioma
synoviosarcoma
synovitis
synovium
Synthes instruments
systemic lupus erythematosus
  (SLE)
sythesis
synthetase
synthetic
syphilis
syringe
syringomyelia

Additional Entries

tabes dorsalis
tabetic
taboparesis
Tachdjiian technique
    (hamstring)
tackler's arm
tactile
tailbone
Tailor's bunion
talar tilt
talipes
    calcanovalgus
    calcaneovarus
    calcaneus
    cavovalgus
    cavus
    equinovalgus
    equinovarus
    equinus
    planovalgus
    valgus
    varus
talocalcaneal
talocalcaneal angle
talocalcaneal coalition
talocrural
talofibular
talonavicular

taloscaphoid
talotibial
talus
Talwin
Tamai technique
tamponade
tangential view
tap
tape
tapered
TARA (total articular
    resurfacing arthroplasty)
tardy nerve palsy
tarsal
tarsal bars
tarsal coalition
tarsal pronator shoes
tarsal tunnel
tarsal tunnel syndrome
tarsalgia
tarsectomy
tarsometatarsal
tarsotarsal
tarsus
TAR syndrome
    (thrombocytopenia-absent
    radius)
Tay-Sachs disease

Additional Entries

Taylor spine brace
Taylor splint (apparatus)
Taylor technique
T-condylar fracture
teardrop fracture
technetium bone scan
technical
technician
technique
TED stockings
Teflon
telangiectasia
teledactyl
telescoping medullary rod
Telfa dressing
temperature
template
tenaculum
tenderness
tendinitis
tendinous
tendolysis
tendon
tendon Achilles lengthening
   (TAL)
tendon reflex
tendon release
tendon transfer
tendonitis
tendosynovitis
tendovaginal

tennis elbow
tennis leg
tennis thumb
tenodesis
tenodynia
tenolysis
tenomyoplasty
tenomyotomy
tenonectomy
tenontagra
tenontodynia
tenontomyoplasty
tenontomyotomy
tenontophyma
tenontoplasty
tenontothecitis
tenophyte
tenoplasty
tenorrhaphy
tenositis
tenostosis
tenosynovectomy
tenosynovitis
tenotomy
TENS (transcutaneous electrical
   nerve stimulator)
tensile
tensile strength
tension
tension band wiring
tensor

Additional Entries

_____
_____
_____
_____
_____
_____
_____
_____
_____

tensor fascia lata
teratocarcinoma
teratogen
teratogenic
teratoma
teres major muscle
teres minor muscle
tertiary
terminal
test
testicle
testosterone
tetanus
tetanic contraction
tetany
Teuffer tendo
  calcaneus repair
tetracaine
tetracycline
Tevdec suture
thalassemia
thallium scan
thalidomide
T-handle reamer
THARIES prosthesis
theatre sign
theca
thenar
thenar eminence
thenar flap
thenar muscles

therapeutic
therapist
therapy
thermal burn
thermal laser
thermogram
thermograph
thermography
thermometer
thermoplastic
thermoregulatory
thiamine
thick split graft
Thiemann disease
Thiersch's graft operation
thigh
thimerosal
thin split graft
thiotepa
third-degree burn
third-degree sprain
third generation (antibiotic)
Thomas heel
Thomas knee splint
Thomas ring
Thomas test
Thomas, Thompson and Straub
  transfer
Thomsen's disease
Thompson approach
Thompson femoral head prosthesis

Additional Entries

Thompson and Compere hip
  arthrodesis
Thompson and Epstein
  classification (hip dislocations)
Thompson and Henry approach
  (humerus)
thoracentesis
thoracic
thoracic outlet syndrome (TOS)
thoroacoacromial
thoracolumbar
thoracometry
thoracomyodynia
thoracoplasty
thoracoscopy
thoracostomy
thoracotomy
thorax
THR (total hip replacement)
thread
threshold
thrill
throbbing
thrombectomy
thrombin
thromboangitis obliterans
thrombocythemia
thrombocytopenia
thromboembolism
thrombolysis
thrombopathy

thrombophlebitis
thromboplastin
thromboplastin time, partial (PPT)
thrombosed
thrombosis
thrombus
thrower's elbow
Thrust femoral prosthesis
thumb
thumb spica
thumb-in-palm deformity
Thurston-Holland's sign
thyroid
tibia
tibia vara
tibial
tibial plateau
tibial tuberosity
tibialis
tibialis anterior
tibialis posterior
tibiocalcaneal
tibiofemoral
tibiofibular
tibiofibular ligament
tibionavicular
tibioperoneal
tibioscaphoid
tibiotalar
tibiotarsal
Ticarcillin

Additional Entries

Ticron suture
t.i.d. (three times a day)
Tietze's syndrome (disease)
Tikhoff-Linberg shoulder girdle
    resection
Tile and Pennal classification
    (pelvic ring fractures)
Tillaux fracture
Tillman resurfacing technique
tilt table
tincture
tincture of iodine
tinea cruris
tinea pedis
Tinel's sign
tingling
tissue
Titan femoral component
titanium
tobramycin
toe
toenail
toe spica
Tohen transfer
Tolectin
tolerance
tolmetin
tomogram
tomography
tone
tongs

tonicity
tonoclonic
tonus
Tooth's atrophy, disease
tophaceous
tophi (pl. of tophus)
tophus
topical
torque
torque heels
torsion
torsional rigidity
torsionometer
torticollis
torus fracture
total ankle
Total articular resurfacing
    arthroplasty (TARA)
total condylar (HSS) knee
    prosthesis
total elbow
total hip replacement (THR)
total knee replacement (TKR)
total shoulder
total wrist
toughness
tourniquet
Townley knee prosthesis
toxemia
toxic
toxicity

Additional Entries

toe-off (refers to walking/gait)

toxin
toxoid
Toxoplasma
toxoplasmosis
trabecula
trabecular
trabecular bone
trabeculation
trace elements
tracer
trachea
tracheostomy
tract
traction
traction bow
traction spur
training
trait
tampoline
tranquilizer
transaxial
transcervical
transcutaneous electrical nerve
   stimulator (TENS)
transducer
transdural
transection
transfix
transfusion
transiliac
transillumination

transischiac
translateral
translation
translocation
translucent
transmissible
transmission
transmitter
transmural
transmutation
transparent
transplant
transplantation
transposition
transpubic
transsection
transthoracic
transudate
transudation
transversalis
transverse
transverse carpal ligament
transverse plane
transverse process
transversectomy
transversotomy
transversus muscle
trapezial
trapeziometacarpal
trapezium
trapezius

Additional Entries

trapezoid
trapezoid bone
trapezoid ligament
Trapezoid total hip prothesis
trauma
traumatic
traumatologist
Trautman Locktite hook
Treacher-Collins syndrome
treadmill test
treatment
tremor
Trendelenburg gait
Trendelenburg sign, test
trephine
threshold
triad
triage
triamcinolone
triangle
triangular fibrocartilage
triangulation technique
triaxial hinge, elbow
triceps
triceps surae muscle
tricepsplasty
trifurcation
trigger digit
trigger finger
trigger finger release
trigger points

trimalleolar fracture
triphalangeal thumb
triplane arthrodesis
triplane fracture
triple arthodesis
triple innominate osteotomy
triplegia
triquetrum
triradial, triradiate
triradiate cartilage
trisomy
trocar
trochanter
trochanteric
trochanterplasty
trochlea
trochlear notch (ulna)
tropocollagen
trough
Tronzo classification
    (trochanteric fractures)
trophic ulcer
Trumble arthrodesis
trunk
truss
tryptophan
T-shaped incision
T-spine
Tsuge technique
Tsuji laminaplasty
tubercle

Additional Entries

tuberculosis
tuberosity
tuberous sclerosis
tubular
tuft
tumefaction
tumor
tumorous
tungsten
tunnel
tunnel view
turbid
Turco technique (clubfoot)

turf toe
turgid
turgor
turnbuckle
turnbuckle cast
Turner's syndrome
turret exostosis
twice a day (BID)
twinge
twitch
two-point discrimination
Tylenol
type and crossmatch (T&C)

Additional Entries

_____
_____
_____
_____
_____
_____
_____
_____
_____
_____
_____
_____
_____
_____
_____
_____
_____
_____
_____
_____
_____
_____
_____
_____
_____
_____

U

UCB orthosis
UCI knee prosthesis
Uematsu shoulder arthrodesis
UHMWPE (ultrahigh molecular weight polyethylene)
ulcer
ulceration
Ullmann's line
ulna
ulnar
ulnar collateral ligament
ulnar deviation
ulnar drift
ulnar tunnel
ulnar tunnel syndrome
ulnar variance
ulnare
ulnaris
ulnocarpal
ulnoradial
ultimate load
ultrasound
ultraviolet light
unbalanced
umbilicus
unconstrained knee prosthesis
unconstrained prosthesis
uncovertebral joint
underarm orthosis
undersized (prosthesis)
undisplaced
uniarticular
unicameral bone cyst
unicompartmental knee implant
unilateral
unilateral bar
union
unipennate muscle
unipolar
unit
Universal exercise equipment
Universal femoral head prosthesis
unmyelinated
Unna's boot
unsegmented bar
ununited
upper extremity
upper motor neuron (UMN)
uptake
urate crystals
Urbaniak technique (hand)
ureter
urethra
urethritis
uric acid
urinalysis

Additional Entries

_____
_____
_____
_____
_____
_____
_____
_____
_____

urinary tract infection (UTI)
urogenital

urogram
urticaria

Additional Entries

V

V-osteotomy
Vac-Pac positioner
vaccine
vacuum
vacumm sign
Vainio arthoplasty
valgus
valgus extension overload
   syndrome
Valium
Valls prothesis
Valpar work test
Valsalva's maneuver
valves
vancomycin
Van Gorder approach
variant
variable resistance exercise
varicose vein
varicosities
varus
varus knee
Vasconez tensor fascia lata flap
vascular
vascular spasm
vascularization
vaseline gauze dressing
vasoconstriction

vasoconstrictor
vasodilatation
vasodilator
vasomoter
vasospasm
vastus intermedius muscle
vastus lateralis muscle
vastus medialis muscle
VDRL test
vector
vein
vein grafts
Velcro splint
Velpeau's bandage
venogram
ventral
venules
Verbrugge bone holding forceps
Verdan graft
Verebelyi-Ogston procedure
verruca plantaris
Versed
vertebra
vertebral body
vertebral column
vertebrectomy
vertebrectomy (Bohlman
   technique)

Additional Entries

vertebrocostal
vertebrosacral
vertical
vertical talus
vertigo
vesicle
vessel
vestigial
viable
vibratory sense
Vicryl suture
villonodular synovitis
   (pigmented)
villus (pl. villi)
villous synovitis
vinblastine sulfate
vincristine sulfate
vinculae
vinculum
vinculum breve
vinculum longum
Vinke tongs
virulent
virus
viscoelastic
viscosity
viscous
vital signs
Vitallium
vitamin

vitamin A
vitamin B
vitamin C
vitamin D
vitamin D-resistant rickets
vitamin E
vitamin supplements
volar
volar flap
volar plate
volar shelf arthroplasty
volar splint
Volkmann's canal, membrane
Volkmann's contracture
voltage
volume
voluntary
Volz elbow hinge
von Langenbeck periosteal
   elevator
VonFrey hair test
von Recklinghausen's disease
von Rosen splint
von Rosen view
von Willebrand's disease (factor
   VIII deficiency)
V-osteotomy
Vulpius-Compere procedure
V-Y muscle-plasty
V-Y plasty

Additional Entries

_____
_____
_____
_____
_____
_____
_____
_____
_____
_____

W

waddling gait
Wadsworth approach (elbow)
Wadsworth hinge
Wagner advancement
Wagner apparatus
Wagner external fixator
Wagner resurfacing technique
Wagner technique (limb lenghtening)
Wagstaffe's fracture
waist
wake-up test
Waldenstrom's disease
Waldenstrom's macroglobulinemia
Walldius knee prosthesis
Wallenbergs syndrome
Wallerian degeneration
walk
Ward's triangle
warfarin
warm-up
Warner and Farber procedure
wart
Wartenburg sign
Wassel's classification (thumb polydactyly)
Watkins spinal fusion

Watson-Cheyne wedge resection
Watson-Jones approach
Watson-Jones arthrodesis
Watson-Jones procedure (ankle)
Waugh knee prosthesis
W.B.C. (white blood cell) count
weaver's bottom
Weaver and Dunn technique
web ligament
web space
web space infection
Weber classification of fractures
Weber and Vasey technique
webbed
webril
Weck knife
wedge
weep
weight bearing
weight lifter's headache (blackout)
weight training
Weiss spring
well-leg traction
Werdnig-Hoffman disease
Werdnig-Hoffman paralysis
WEST (work evaluation systems technology)

Additional Entries

West and Soto-Hall procedure
Wet Bulb Globe Temperature
   Index (WBGT)
wet-bulb temperature
wet-to-dry dressing
wet reading
wheelchair
wind chill factor
whiplash
whirlpool bath
White procedure
Whiteside prosthesis
Whitesides and Kelly approach
whitlow (herpetic)
Whitman technique
Whitman and Thompson
   procedure
Whitman frame
Whitman osteotomy
Whitman plate
Whitman talectomy procedure
Whitman's operation
whole blood
Wiberg shelf procedure
Wickstrom arthrodesis
Wilkin's classification (radial
   neck fractures)
Williams flexion exercises
Williams orthosis
Williams and Haddad procedure
Wilmington jacket

Wilms' tumor
Wilson technique
Wilson and Jacobs procedure
Wilson and McKeever procedure
Wilson approach
Wilson graft
Wilson plate
Winberger line
windlass, Spanish
window
windshield wiper sign
Winquist and Hansen
   classification (femoral
   fractures)
Winter anterior osteotomy
wire
wiring
Wirth and Jager posterior
   cruciate reconstruction
within normal limits (WNL)
Wolf procedure
Wolfe skin graft
Wolfe-Kawamoto iliac graft
Wolfe-Krause graft
Wolff's law
Woodward elevation of scapula
work evaluation systems
   technology (WEST)
work hardening program
workout
wormian bone

Additional Entries

woven bone
wound
W-plasty
wraparound dressing
Wright knee prosthesis
wringer injury

Wrisberg-ligament
wrist
wristdrop
wryneck
wt. (weight)

Additional Entries

Wy bunionectomy

Additional Entries

X

xanthoma   xiphoid
xenograft   x-linked
Xeroform dressing x-ray
xerogram

Additional Entries

Additional Entries

Y

Y fracture
YAG laser
Y incision
Y-line
Y-osteotomy

Yee approach
Yergason test
yield stress
Young approach
Young procedure

Additional Entries

Additional Entries

Z

Zadik procedure
Zancolli capsulodesis
Zancolli technique
Zarins and Rowe procedure
Zeir procedure
Zenotech
Zephiran
Zickel nail
zig-zag incision

Zimmerman's pericytes
Zinacef
zinc
zinc oxide
Z line (muscle)
Zorprin
Z-plasty
Zuelzer hook plate
Zyloprim

Additional Entries

Notes:
   Compression sleeves are placed
on the unaffected side after some
~~other~~ ortho surgeries for
DVT prophylaxis.